A Systems-Centered Approach
to Inpatient Group Psychotherapy

of related interest

Autobiography of a Theory
Developing Systems-Centered Theory
Yvonne M. Agazarian and Susan P. Gantt
ISBN 1 85302 847 9

The Group as Therapist
Rachael Chazan
International Library of Group Analysis 14
ISBN 1 85302 906 8

The Evolution of Group Analysis
Edited by Malcolm Pines
International Library of Group Analysis 16
ISBN 1 85302 925 4

Foundations and Applications of Group Psychotherapy
A Sphere of Influence
Mark F. Ettin
International Library of Group Analysis 10
ISBN 1 85302 795 2

Taking the Group Seriously
Towards a Post-Foulkesian Group Analytic Theory
Farhad Dalal
International Library of Group Analysis 5
ISBN 1 85302 642 5

A Systems-Centered Approach to Inpatient Group Psychotherapy

Yvonne M. Agazarian

Jessica Kingsley Publishers
London and Philadelphia

First published in the United Kingdom in 2001 by
Jessica Kingsley Publishers Ltd
116 Pentonville Road
London N1 9JB, England
and
325 Chestnut Street
Philadelphia, PA 19106, USA

www.jkp.com

Library of Congress Cataloging in Publication Data
A CIP catalog record for this book is available from the Library of Congress

British Library Cataloguing in Publication Data
A CIP catalogue record for this book is available from the British Library

ISBN 1 85302 917 3

Printed and Bound in Great Britain by
Athenaeum Press, Gateshead, Tyne and Wear

Contents

List of Figures and Tables

Figures

Tables

Acknowledgements

Great gratitude to the people whose pioneering maps guided my way: Wilfred Bion, John Bowlby, Harold Bridger, Warren Bennis and Herb Shepard, Habib Davanloo, Helen Durkin, Sigmund Freud, Hanna Greenburg, Alan Howard and Robert Scott, Melanie Klein, Alfred Korzybski, Kurt Lewin, Claude Shannon and Warren Weaver, Edwin Schroedinger, Dave Jenkins, George Vassiliou, Ludwig von Bertalanffy.

Great gratitude to the people who helped me to revise my map: all the weekly training groups – specially Friday Group; all the group members (trainees and patients) who have worked with me through the transition from psychoanalysis to group-as-a-whole to systems-centered training and therapy; specially the groups on Monday, Wednesday and Thursday and in New York. Also the SCT centers in Austin, Boston, York and Copenhagen and the Institute Committee of the American Group Psychotherapy Association.

Great gratitude to my friends who were the containing environment for my work: Anne Alonso, Donald Brown, Claudia Byram, Jay Fidler, Fran Carter, Ken Eisold, Susan Gantt, Leonard Horwitz, Anita Simon, Berj Philibossian, Malcolm Pines.

Introduction

This book is about the changing reality in the world of mental health and it is written for those who are responsible for guiding the change. The changes that are addressed are not only those that we are learning to make in the new environment for our practice: this book also introduces the change that systems-centered thinking introduces in the hope that it may be useful in reconceptualizing our ways of doing therapy.

Since the revolution in the world of mental health of the 1990s, one of the experiences which I (and perhaps you too) am constantly both enraged and challenged by is the process of re-orienting myself from long-term to short-term therapy and recognizing that most of the ways I had clinically practiced, supervised and taught, no longer fit.

In the US, health management organizations (HMOs) introduced the values of cost-effective business which collided with the therapist's concern for the therapeutic rhythm that is required for deep change. Business organizations are aware that 'time is money.' Therefore HMOs in the US are inevitably oriented towards their 'product' (outcome): symptom remission and a return to social functioning.

To those of us who are used to taking whatever time the therapy seems to need, the three, five or ten sessions typically allocated for a treatment plan are a big challenge, and there is hardly time to tell whether or not it is at the expense of therapeutic insight. Shared jokes help a little – like the one about the HMO executive who arrived at the pearly gates and was greeted by St Peter: 'Welcome to heaven, I am authorized to give you three days.'

HMOs introduced conflict. I, like others who had seen patients as often as three to five times a week, expected to work with them for as long as it took, even though it took five or ten years, or more. I, like others who were analytically and psychodynamically oriented, was aware that the cost of intensive treatment for the patient was not just in terms of time and money – our own training analysis had required a lot of both. The cost also lay in the intense transference relations that do not remain confined to the therapeutic hour, so that the patient's relationship to therapy could all too easily become more important than his or her relationships at home.

I brought these concerns as a clinician into a changing world. I shared with other therapists the experience of being intensely enraged, bewildered, disheartened and challenged. As I write, I recognize that it was the very intensity of my experience that fueled my next steps. That being challenged to think about my field in terms of short-term therapy, I turned to putting the theory of living human systems into practice. From this, I developed systems-centered therapy for both short-term and long-term therapy.

My major breakthrough came when I understood how to think about short-term therapy in a way that maintained the integrity and values of our work. The solution was to make every therapeutic session a therapy in itself on the one hand, and a step in a hierarchy of steps that would end in meeting all the realistic treatment goals for the *persons* of patient and therapist. Thus, whether a person came for one session, or for as many as it takes, each session would address the particular therapeutic step that the patient could take in the journey towards mental health.

The central theme of this book is how these methods looked when I tried them out with inpatients. It is written around the work of nine inpatients of mixed diagnosis who volunteered to work with me for an hour-and-a-half video-taped group therapy session. As you follow the interactions between me and them, you will get a picture of what the first session of a systems-centered therapy group is like. I will also discuss with you why I did what I did, where what I did fits in terms of the methods and techniques of systems-centered therapy, how it differs from psychodynamic therapy in practice (perhaps more in its approach than its goals), and also how it translates the ideas about living human systems into the real world of people in therapy.

Thus I speak to you of three different aspects of experience in our field today. Perhaps you who read this will find that all three speak to your experience, or perhaps one or other of these aspects speak directly to you.

1. First, I speak to those of you who are entering a new field (or whose old field has suddenly become new) and who are having to fly by the seat of your pants; also, to those who look for guidelines and find them either incomprehensible or out of date; and to those who are not comforted by the fact that many of the clinicians you work with are also in a 'new' field. To you I give many examples of how systems-centered practice looks and sounds in the real world of therapy so that you have a better chance of recognizing it when you see it and deciding whether or not you want to learn how to do it.

2. Second, I speak to those of you who have had many years of experience in long-term therapy in the field and have been confronted with how you are going to adapt your skills to this new short-term therapy world. I introduce a method that applies to both short-term and long-term therapy that is not a compromise. I compare and contrast the

methods of the psychodynamic approach with those of the systems-centered approach, and emphasize that though the systems-centered methods are certainly different they address the same underlying dynamics and share the same goals. These goals are to make the unconscious conscious and to increase the ability of the patients to contain their impulses, conflicts and emotions so that they are less compelled to act out or repeat and more able to use their insight to address the realities of their lives.

3. Third, I speak to those who have always been interested in why things work and who have found that the explanations outlined in the literature do not explain enough – for you, I have written a chapter on theory. The relationship between the theory of living human systems and its systems-centered practice is summarized in a chart (p.134) (I).

The heart of this book

The heart of this book is the verbatim script of a video-taped session with nine inpatients who worked with me in an experimental group, testing out whether or not systems-centered methods would be useful to the more compromised patients. It was the first time I had used the methods and techniques of my systems-centered approach with an inpatient population, and my heart was in my mouth. The session was video-taped and then transcribed. This word by word reproduction of the group is used, in this book, to illustrate what the systems-centered approach is like in real life. The script will give you a very good picture of how functional subgrouping is introduced in a beginning group as the context in which the first three defenses in the SCT (systems-centered therapy) hierarchy of defense modification are addressed.

Before reading further, it may be helpful to readers to have a map of how to find their way around this book. Immediately following this introduction, in Chapter One, there is an overview of systems-centered ideas and how they came to be put into practice. Chapter Two is the verbatim script taken from the video-tape of the hour-and-a-half meeting where the inpatient group and I worked together. Wherever there is an opportunity to see an event through my eyes, or to think through, with me, the SCT rationale for a particular intervention, a paragraph of commentary interrupts the script. Readers may prefer to skip these and simply stay with the rhythm of the script, and return for the commentaries afterwards if they wish. Chapter Three discusses the techniques that were used with the group, and revisits many aspects of the script as illustrations of the thinking behind the interventions. Chapter Four is written for those of you who are interested in theory and enjoy wrestling with it. It is not a necessary chapter for any of you who find theory a chore as Chapter One provides a sufficient presentation and discussion of the methods that were developed for SCT and the theoretical constructs they defined. The presentation of the script and the techniques that influenced the course of the group are also sufficient to get a feel for systems-centered therapy without having to know its theoretical roots, unless you wish to.

Orientation to the Systems-Centered Perspective

Let me start by telling you a true story. One sunny summer day in 1983, I was lunching with my friend George Vassiliou in his garden in Athens. We were talking about applying general systems theory to group psychotherapy. To illustrate a point, George threw a piece of his hamburger into the goldfish pond. One goldfish, faster than the others, reached the hamburger first. It was too large for him to swallow, and he swam off with it in his jaws, while the other goldfish darted around him, nibbling away at his prize.

George pointed to the goldfish with the meat in his mouth. 'That poor little fellow is having his dinner stolen from him by the other fish, and if he is not careful, he will have nothing left to eat but the last small bite.'

On the other hand, said George, you might think, here is a whole shoal of fish with a large meal falling into its midst. It is too big a serving for any single fish, so one fish holds it while others nibble away at it and the rest dart after the bits that drift away into the water. Thus all the fish are fed (Agazarian 1989b).

This story illustrates two perspectives on the same event. When we observe a goldfish pond, it makes no difference to the fish whether we say: 'The individual fish has had all his dinner nibbled away except the last bite,' or 'The shoal has developed an efficient food distribution center.'

However, saying to a group the equivalent of 'This poor little fellow is having his lunch stolen from him by the rest of you' will have a very different impact from saying 'You are solving the problem of how to feed your whole population from one otherwise indigestible lump of hamburger.' One could expect the reactions, subsequent events, and even, perhaps, the future course of the group to be significantly influenced by which of the two interpretations one makes.

A theory of living human systems and its systems-centered practice

First let me introduce you to the extra dimension in the goldfish pond that a theory of living human systems adds to general systems theory (von Bertalanffy 1969). General systems theory has already contributed the dimension of the shoal as well as that of the individual fish.

A theory of living human systems introduces a third dimension to the systems of 'shoal' and its 'members.' It adds the system of subgroups (Agazarian 1989a, 1992). First, there is the shoal-as-a-whole perspective, which allows one to watch the shoal as a system. Watching the shoal as a dynamic system, one sees how it has structured itself and how it is functioning: a shoal of fish, separated into two distinct clusters, with some fish crossing randomly from one cluster to another. As systems-centered thinkers we immediately frame the clusters as 'subgroups,' subgroups which exist in the environment of the shoal, and are the environment for its subgroup members. This is a very important frame for us as it allows us to see any system as having three components, and to talk about groups of people in terms of the systems of members, subgroups and the group-as-a-whole. Which dimension we observe will depend upon what we are looking for (Agazarian and Janoff 1993).

For example, if we are interested in individual fish, we will watch the different fish in three different contexts. How we understand the fishes' behavior will change as we shift our attention to the different contexts, just as our under-standing changed when we thought about the hamburger fish in the role of victim or the role of distributor. We can identify how the roles change when we think of the fish in a subgroup context – the cluster that is releasing the bits of hamburger into the water and the cluster that is darting around eating it. And when we think of the fish in the context of the shoal-as-a-whole, we can observe either an individual fish as it moves from one cluster to another and wonder what meaning his movement has from his individual perspective, or wonder what meaning it has for the shoal-as-a-whole, or both. This is how one comes to think of an individual member as a voice for the self and also a voice for the group.

From the group-as-a-whole perspective we can think in exactly the same way about subgroups: what meaning do the subgroups have for the group-as-a-whole, and what meaning does each subgroup have in terms of itself? Systems are isomorphic (similar in structure and function) so whenever we want to we can apply the same kind of thinking (as we just did) to all the different levels in the hierarchy. This is very important to systems-centered thinking as it allows us to think about individual people as systems that have the same three dimensions that we have defined for groups: a person-as-a-whole system which contains subgroup systems, and a member system which can join any one of the internal subgroups at different times. Everyone has membership in many subgroups, but one can only work in one subgroup at a time. Individual people can not only take membership inside their personal selves, but they can also take up membership in a group. The ideal, of course, is for the person to choose which subgroup inside themselves they want to learn more about and then join a subgroup in the group that is exploring the same issues.

It may be an unfamiliar idea that one can deliberately choose which subgroup inside oneself to take membership in. Let me illustrate this by using the analogy of the ego, id and super-ego, and frame them as three subsystems of the person system. You will notice that each has a different function and each has a different and recognizable language (system output). The ego system can be defined as an observing, information collecting system whose language tends to be data oriented. The super-ego system can be defined as a judging system, whose language contains injunctions based upon interpretations, either of how reality should be, or how reality is. The id can be defined as the system containing the life force and whose language communicates want (typically in one syllable words).

From this analogy, framing the ego, super-ego and id as functions that have predictable communications (information outputs), it can be seen that it is possible to diagnose in which subgroup inside themselves the person has taken up membership. Similarly it will be possible to listen to the different languages in the group, identify which subgroups are present and which members belong to each. There are two important aspects of framing group dynamics this way. First it becomes possible to identify the group's subgroups by analyzing the communication (a group process variable). Second there is a clear discrimination between process and content – two subgroups may have the same content but process it in very different ways. Third, it becomes clear that the way a person takes up membership in internal subgroups has the potential for linking directly into the group subgroups, either implicitly or explicitly.

Framing subgroups in this way allows the therapist to understand and intervene into aspects of group dynamics that they might have difficulty understanding without identifying the implicit subgroups. For example, a group that has split into super-ego and id subgroups is more likely to act out than a group that has split into super-ego and ego subgroups. A simple intervention might make a big difference to the acting out potential if the therapist encourages the super-ego subgroup to discriminate between relating to what *is* rather than what *ought to be.*

A theory of living human systems (TLHS)

A theory of living human systems defines a hierarchy of isomorphic systems that are energy-organizing, self-correcting and goal-oriented (Agazarian 1997).

In the discussion above I have used the goldfish analogy to define the hierarchy for systems-centered therapy: member, subgroup and group-as-a-whole. In the paragraphs that follow, I talk more about these systems. Theory is constructed of words (like building blocks), each of which must have a specific definition which, ideally, makes some intuitive sense.

Hierarchy of systems

In a systems-centered hierarchy it is assumed that each system exists in the environment of the system above it and is the environment of the system below it. When we apply this to the goldfish pond we have the subgroups that exist in the environment of the shoal and are the environment for their members.

Member systems are represented by the individual goldfish who are members of the shoal. The member systems exist in the environment (or context) of the subgroups (clusters) in the context of the system 'shoal' (the group-as-a-whole).

Subgroup systems are represented by two clusters of goldfish: the cluster that is competing for the hamburger and the more widely spread cluster of goldfish who are chasing the bits that are floating away. The subgroup systems exist in the environment (or context) of the group-as-a-whole. One has to develop an eye for identifying subgroups. If one did not observe that the bits of hamburger are being released into the water by the activity of the fish that are nibbling at it, one might not recognize that both the nibbling fish and the hamburger chasing fish are two complementary subgroups achieving the system-as-a-whole goal of food distribution among the population.

The group-as-a-whole system is represented by the shoal with its implicit goal of food distribution. When one can see the hamburger as an explicit group goal that both the member fish and the subgroups are relating to, it is also possible to intuit the implicit goal of the system, which is to survive as a system through distributing food to itself. (We assume that living human systems have three implicit goals: to survive, to develop and to transform from simpler to more complex.)

The most familiar perspective to us is the personal perspective, the person system. From the personal perspective we can become aware that any single event has as many meanings as we have contexts for it. However, that is only when we do not take things just personally. When we take things 'just personally' we lose all other contexts except our own. A major goal in systems-centered therapy is to enable the members to develop a 'researcher' that enables them to test experience from the different contexts of member, subgroup, group-as-a-whole for both themselves and the group. What we are discovering, as our group members have put this into practice, is that taking things 'just' personally seems to be the major source of human anguish – and although the event does not alter, altering the perspective changes the experience from unbearable anguish to bearable reality.

Contextualizing

Developing one's 'researcher' develops an observing system (in the person system) whose function is to discriminate and integrate information. Developing the observing self-system is the first step in the method called contextualizing. Contextualizing is the operational definition of hierarchy. Contextualizing deliberately brings into the minds of people who join a systems-centered group the idea of the member, the subgroup and the group-as-a-whole (discrimination). Once this idea is understood, the mind is then open to understanding that as the context changes not only does the experience change, but also the responsibilities of taking up the role that is specific to the goals of the context. In other words, as a member of one's person, the goal is to bridge between membership in oneself into membership in the group (integration). This is almost certainly isomorphic to all contexts. In the context of a systems-centered group it is spelled out as a social responsibility. The goal of 'member' in the context of an SCT group is to join, authentically, the subgroup of the self with a subgroup of the group.

The goal of the subgroup is to explore one side of group conflict as deeply as is natural to the subgroup, until the issues are integrated in the group-as-a-whole. The goal of the group-as-a-whole is to contain the dynamics, either in functional subgrouping or, when the group is not in conflict, in the work of the group-as-a-whole. Containing is a boundarying goal. The functional goal is for the system hierarchy to survive, develop and transform from simpler to more complex through the process of discriminating and integrating differences.

Discovering subgroups

In thinking theory, in the process of trying to make a connection between the idea and the real world I (like many other theoreticians) rely on a transitional step of illustrating ideas, or doodling. My doodles are usually arrows and circles. The definition of hierarchy was easy to intuit by three concentric circles, the center one for member, the outside one for the group-as-a-whole and the middle one for subgroup. Mulling over these three circles and wondering what they might mean in reality, the implication suddenly hit me. If the subgroup existed in the environment of the group-as-a-whole, and if the subgroup was the environment for its members, then the subgroup, which shared its boundaries with both of the other two, was the central system of the three.

The implications were startling. I had always taken it for granted that the individual was the basic unit of the group. But looking at these three circles, the basic unit of groups was not the individual member (as in patient-centered groups), not the leader (as in leader-centered groups), and not the group itself (as in group-as-a-whole-centered groups), but the subgroup. Thus I had introduced a fourth orientation to the other three: systems-centered groups in which the basic unit was the subgroup. If the subgroup was indeed the basic unit of the group, then influencing the subgroup would be more functional than influencing either the person or the group-as-a-whole. This was fine in theory, but I had no idea how to test it in practice.

The first step towards understanding how to reframe my thinking came when I remembered the panel at the American Group Psychotherapy Association (AGPA) in which we had all analyzed the same video-tape of a 'difficult' patient group which was to be discussed from four different therapeutic modalities, mine being the modality of Tavistock[1] and the group-as-a-whole. I remembered that I had written (without fully understanding what I was saying) that subgroups are not defined by individual people! (Agazarian 1987). At that time I was demonstrating how group members were a voice for both themselves and the group and later used the same episode when I was introducing the idea of subgroups (Agazarian 1989). This is a good example of how I did not hear my own voice until I was able to change the context.

The video-tape starts with a knock on the door. Then a late patient, Bess, enters and there is much commotion as everybody makes room and squashes their chairs together. The dialogue goes like this:

Therapist 1 (a nurse): Fine, come on in...

Therapist 2 (a resident): Why don't you...here, take this chair...

Therapist 1: Watch the wire...

Bess: Yeah...

Alice: Move the table...

Edna: The camera will break...

(*Alice, Bess, Clark, Edna, Doris, Glenda laugh*)

Alice: It's called togetherness (*as they all squash their chairs together*)

Clark: Closeness...

Bess: That's what we're all looking for...

Therapist: All thinking...

Therapist 2: Ready?...

Alice: Christmas...

Therapist 2: We were just talking about the fact that Edna was seeing me individually for treatment of her depression...

My group-as-a-whole orientation had trained me to hear how each member was a voice, not only for themselves, but also for the group (Agazarian and Peters 1981). It was while I was analyzing the script that I discovered that members' voices also defined the group's subgroups, and that these subgroups were not formal (like therapists and patients) but functional as they carried a voice for potential work important to the group.

As I listened to the tape again, I heard a duet between two subgroups, one giving voice about how to structure the group, the other giving voice about the yearning for intimacy.

Structuring subgroup:

'Here, sit here.'

'Take this chair'

'Don't trip over the wire.'

'Move the table.'

'Come on in.'

'Ready?'

Togetherness subgroup:

'Come on in.'

'It's called togetherness.'

'Closeness.'

'That's what we're all looking for.'

'That's what we're all thinking.'

'It's like Christmas.'

Functionally, these two subgroups had come into being around two separate themes: managing the group boundaries and the yearning for 'togetherness.' They were not determined by individual people (Alice's voice, for example, is heard in both subgroups) nor by role (both patients and the therapist contributed to both subgroups). It was also clear that the therapists could not respond to the 'togetherness' theme (which would be central work for the group) if they did not hear it. In fact, sadly enough, the response 'We were just talking about the fact that Edna was seeing me individually for treatment of her depression' turned the group away from 'togetherness' towards competition, jealousy and envy, which may have belonged more to the therapist's agenda than the patients'.

As soon as I recognized the subgroups, I found myself deeply moved. I had a new and deeper sense of what I thought I already knew – that the dynamics of group were as profound and real as the dynamics of individuals, and contained whole dimensions of meaning that one could not hear if one listened only to the individual members.

It is not a new idea, of course, that subgroups emerge spontaneously in a group. It was new to me, however, to see that there was implicit as well as explicit subgrouping. I could see a big difference between recognizing how explicitly members come together around stereotype similarities (like race, religion, gender, politics and status) and discovering how members spontaneously join around underlying group themes (as in the 'togetherness' subgroup above).

Subgrouping in a group is typically implicit rather than explicit. It is rare in a group to have someone say explicitly 'Let's divide the group up into black and white, or young and old, or high status, low status.' Spontaneous subgrouping around stereotyping, however, does occur with great frequency in groups and is one of the ways that groups implicitly (and unwittingly) organize themselves. The advantage is the group stabilizes itself around the familiar. The cost is that building alliances based on stereotypes is rarely the best way of bringing members' resources together for the work that the group has come to do. In addition, structuring a group around social stereotyping tends to set up we/they tensions which often lead to scapegoating.

Another type of implicit subgrouping occurs when members come together, not around familiar stereotypes, but around a defense (like Bion's (1959) flight or fight) or around a common theme – sometimes goal-related work, and sometimes not.

It was the process of discovering these underlying subgroup dynamics and making them explicit to the groups that I was leading that the groups became able to choose what they wanted to subgroup around. This was a gigantic step towards developing SCT's functional subgrouping, in which members are explicitly asked to join on the similarities that they resonate with.

Later, as functional subgrouping developed in greater complexity, it was to emerge as a conflict resolution technique in which integration takes place through an explicit subgrouping process which contains the different sides of the conflict in the group-as-a-whole rather than in its members (Agazarian 1997). Each member is free to choose the subgroup that represents best the side of the conflict he or she wishes to explore first. In untrained groups, learning how to subgroup comes before deliberately using it to contain and resolve conflict. In the inpatient unit script in Chapter Two, subgrouping is still in the early stages of development.

In my work so far, however much I had drawn patients' attention to the group, my observations led me to believe that their major transferential relationships were with me, not each other. My data was that group members worked with one eye on each other and the other eye on me. It goes without saying that I was concerned that this constant revectoring of work energy away from me and back into the subgroup might be too painful for some (if not all) group members. In the early days of Tavistock, when therapists interpreted only to the group-as-a-whole, many patients felt dehumanized and discounted (Yalom, Liebermann and Miles 1973[2]). In response to these research results I had earlier modified my group-as-a-whole technique by looking at members directly if the group-as-a-whole intervention had a specific relevance to them.

Built into the roles of doctor and patient is the one-up/one-down relationship[3] that so easily provokes childhood transference. I had been interested, for many years, in finding ways of working with groups that laid more emphasis on building the kind of group society that, rather than increasing the pressure to act out in response to the group dynamics, in itself contributed to containing and exploring the underlying dynamics by making them less, rather than more, threatening. Pat de Maré (de Maré, Piper and Thompson 1991) had relied on the variable of group size. I had been looking for variables that were independent of the size of the group.

The first step was to turn the group's eyes away from me and into their subgroup. In the process of developing SCT, I was to learn that this triangulation by eye contact occurred predominantly in the early phases of group development, most strongly in the first subphase of flight, less in the subphase of fight, and only as a group-as-a-whole focus on me as the object of group disappointment in the difficult subphase of resistance to change.

Now, as we in SCT promote functional subgrouping in a beginning group, we legitimize and make explicit the conflict between looking towards the therapist or looking towards the subgroup by saying something like: 'Do you notice that you have one eye on me and one eye on your subgroup? Almost everybody does at this stage of group development (normalizing)[4]. This puts you at a fork in the road – a choice. You can explore the conflict between being pulled towards your relationship with me, your therapist, or you can explore your relationship to the subgroup you are working in.' When triangulation becomes available as a group issue, then the group-as-a-whole can subgroup around being pulled in two directions at once. Managing responses to eye contact in this way is an example of making early manifestations of the underlying, transferential issues around dependency accessible at a level that the group is able to work.

This is a good example of how a natural group dynamic (like keeping an eye on the leader) is good material for functional subgrouping. Rather than being an embarrassment for an SCT group, it becomes a challenge to identify and explore the conflict. Almost certainly it will be framed by the group as a choice between the impulse to depend on the leader and the impulse to pull away and relate to each other. Thus, quite early in the group process, the group is exploring dependency in the containing environment of a subgroup, and as deeply as the subgroup can go, rather than experiencing the embarrassment, shame or guilt that so often accompanies this work.

Functional subgrouping is the basic systems-centered process which requires people to come together and explore their similarities instead of stereotyping or scapegoating their differences. As members explore their experience in the comfortably cohesive climate of similarity, attunement and resonance of their subgroup, they are able to become aware of their differences as well as their similarities. Thus, in the process of recognizing and integrating differences within the subgroup, human similarities (that were previously denied) become apparent between the different subgroups. As similarities between the apparently different subgroups are recognized, integration takes place in the group-as-a-whole.

The technique of functional subgrouping had done more than introduce a method of working with discrimination and integration of information. The very process that subgroup members used to explore their experience on a journey of discovery without interpretive guidance from the therapist allowed me, as the therapist, the luxury of observing the discoveries that members made at deeper and deeper levels of dynamics. (Also, without the terror that so often accompanies the patients and analysands into their unconscious – the subgroup is a very different holding environment from the couch.) My experience was like sitting in on a course in group and individual dynamics given by teachers who were discovering as they taught. When, as an analyst, I had sat behind the couch, I had the psychoanalytic frame in which to interpret the dynamics. In contrast, my frame in my beginning work as an SCT therapist was arrows and circles. In SCT, my understanding literally came from noticing the differences in what was apparently similar to what I knew and discovering new kinds of similarities in those differences.

I was also able to contrast norms that were established in the groups with functional subgrouping with the norms that were established by stereotype subgrouping. It became clear that each phase and subphase of group development were characterized by particular kinds of stereotypic subgrouping and specific kinds of defensive communications generic to each phase. By substituting functional subgrouping for stereotype subgrouping, groups moved into and out of each phase without some of the acting out that I had come to take for granted as characteristic of most (if not all) groups. For example, groups rarely set up identified patients or scapegoats when members explored their impulses in functional subgroups rather than acting them out. It was in this way that the norms that identify systems-centered groups were established.

The systems-centered group

From the first few seconds of a systems-centered group the therapist introduces the SCT vocabulary and the methods which establish the characteristic norms of an SCT group. These norms are brought into being by four specific methods that make the bridge between theory and practice (Agazarian 1997). The group structure is influenced through boundarying interventions. The group process is influenced through functional subgrouping interventions. The group goal direction is influenced through vectoring interventions. The establishment of a system hierarchy is influenced through contextualizing interventions that develop awareness of how each system (member and subgroup and group-as-a-whole) has goals that differ from each other and are different again from the individual system.

In the process of developing these methods, some challenging questions arose. For example, as all systems in the hierarchy are defined as isomorphic (similar in structure and function), would all the systems in the hierarchy be influenced if one influenced either the structure or the function of any one? It seemed so. Modifying the communicating pattern in either member, subgroup or group-as-a-whole did appear to influence the norms of communicating at all system levels.

The hierarchy of systems is defined by three systems: the member system, subgroup system and system-as-a-whole. As the subgroup exists in the environment of the system-as-a-whole and is the environment for its members, would it be more effective to influence the subgroup rather than either the member or the group-as-a-whole? It seems that it was. Introducing functional subgrouping as an alternative to stereotype subgrouping made it easier for the group and its members to connect to the work goals.

This led to a further question. If this hierarchy is applied both to individuals as systems and groups as systems, would this make both group responses and individual responses less predictable? It seemed that it would. In the real world, the person that enters the group is the 'raw material' from which a systems-centered member and the systems-centered group is developed. As people learn to take on the role of the systems-centered member in relationship to the subgroups of the group-as-a-whole, they also learn to take on a role in relationship to their own internal subgroups of their person-as-whole. The person-as-a-whole is an idea at one end of the abstraction ladder, with the real person at the other end, who has personal experiences when he or she enters into a new group as a potential member. It is membership that is the link between the group and the individual, and it is in the person-as-a-whole that group insight is integrated. Becoming aware of experience as a member of the group-as-a-whole and its subgroups increases the potential for insight in more than one context, and also formally introduces the discrimination between personal experience and personalizing. By personalizing (taking things 'just' personally), the person is only aware of themselves as the context, self-centered at the expense of being 'systems-centered.'

Another question arises from the assumption that all living human systems survive, develop and transform through the process of discriminating and integrating differences. Did this mean that the typical responses to group conflict would change if individuals and groups were required to address conflict by discriminating and integrating the differences that are causing the conflict? It seemed so. Membership in functional subgroup work in the group enabled both the group and the individual to integrate differences which otherwise would have been targeted or ignored. A major surprise was to discover that scapegoating, that

I had always taken for granted as an unavoidable phase in the life of groups, was explored instead of acted out in systems-centered groups.

Contextualizing, boundarying, subgrouping and vectoring

So far in this chapter I have traced the history of the discovery of functional subgrouping because, of all the methods that have been generated from a theory of living human systems (Agazarian 1997), it is probably the one that will generalize most easily into groups , whether or not they are 'systems-centered.' It is, however, only one of four methods that were developed from the theory and put into practice in systems-centered therapy. These four methods are: contextualizing (the operational definition of hierarchy); boundarying (the operational definition of isomorphy of structure); functional subgrouping (the operational definition of the isomorphy of function); and vectoring (the operational definition of the energy that fuels the living human system's ability to be self-correcting, energy-organizing and goal-directed) (see endnote 6).

I will introduce each of these four methods briefly in the paragraphs below as an orientation to systems-centered practice. How they apply in a real group is demonstrated with the verbatim script of the inpatient unit group which met with me for one session as an experiment to see how SCT methods would work with inpatients (see Chapter Two).

Boundarying

Isomorphy, in a theory of living human systems, means that systems in the defined hierarchy are isomorphic: that is, similar in structure and function. This requires two definitions: one for structure, one for function. I have already discussed the operational definition for function in the paragraphs above about functional subgrouping. Structure, which will be discussed below, is defined in terms of boundaries that exist in space and time: both geographical space and clock time, and the psychological boundaries between the past, future, and the present awareness of the self in relationship outside and inside the group.

From the systems-centered perspective, the boundaries of treatment are defined by the context. For therapists who do not frame group dynamics within the context of phases of group development, there are only two contexts available: the individual as a context and the group as a context. What is not available to group therapists who see only individuals in the group is the existence of the person in the context of the subgroup and also in the context of the group-as-a-whole. Without context, there is no clear understanding that the influence of the psychological environment will have just as much impact as the physical environment.

Thinking of 'individual,' 'subgroup' and 'group' as three 'systems' in a hierarchy of related systems requires an additional discipline of thinking (Agazarian and Janoff 1993), but one which does not contradict the existing body of psychodynamic knowledge. In fact, SCT draws heavily upon psychodynamics when it comes to the application of the theory in practice. A systems perspective, however, does provide an additional way of looking at the dynamics of the individual, the subgroup and the group, so that the combined understanding of group and individual dynamics can be applied to the practice of group psychotherapy. The additional dimension that systems thinking introduces is what I would call 'complementarity.'

Complementarity is a basic orientation in systems thinking. Like yin/yang, it describes the principle of always being separate but always related. In SCT thinking, things are thought about in terms of either/or only when it is useful to dichotomize.

For example, when thinking about group psychotherapy, it is true that as the person matures, so the person interacts more maturely with the group, and as the member interactions mature so does the group-as-a-whole. It is also true that as the group-as-a-whole matures, increased maturity is required of its members.

The method of boundarying not only determines the structure of the real group in real space and time, but is also aimed at influencing the boundary permeability to information by reducing the noise in the communication process. The theory of living human systems (TLHS) assumes that systems open their boundaries to clear communication and close their boundaries to noise. This was a very important theoretical definition in the development of SCT. It simply turned upside down the approach that I had always used in group therapy, which was to *follow* the group while it found its own way towards some kind of valid communication. The implications, however, were inescapable. The more noise that enters the group, the more difficult it will be for the group to enter into clear communication and the more difficult it will be for the members to do their work. It seemed more practical to attempt to filter out the noise *before* it crossed the boundary into the group, and to clear up the noise *as soon as* it arose in the group. Noisy communication is defensive communications that are accepted as familiar ways of talking like social chatter, being vague, telling stories and keeping distance with a 'yes' followed by a 'but.' Deciding to change accepted communication norms from the first few minutes of a group meant that I had to change the way that I had always led groups. I had to change from active listening to active intervention. In a surprisingly short time, I found that when I heard defensive communications, they served as a signal for me to interrupt as soon as I heard them. For example, 'because' almost always continues into an explanation, and 'yes, but' almost always pre-empts the other person's point of view. Introducing interrupting as a type of intervention posed a challenge: How to intervene in such a way that it would sufficiently peak the members' curiosity so that the interruptions were experienced as a therapeutic intervention? The solution seemed to be to nest the interruptions in facts that could be checked by the member and that made sense to him or her.

It took many hours of patient supervisory help for me to make the transition from the active listening of the psychodynamic and analytic approach to the active intervention of the systems-centered approach and to learn to ask explicitly rather than to interpret silently. An example is in my response to Rose when she joined the oppositional subgroup:

> Rose: I don't know if I would term it that I am waiting to have a feeling.
>
> YA: How would you term it?

Passing the ball to the patient with 'How would you term it?' required a total shift in the way I took up my therapist role. In my psychodynamic therapist role, before I learned active intervention, I would pay attention to the meaning of the patient's transference resistance to me; what connections I could make between her present responses and past experiences; whether I judged her reaction to have more to do with her relationship with her mother or her father; and what could I learn from my own counter-transference reaction. (In relationship to Rose I had a counter-transference response of being instantly on the alert – as if I had suddenly come on sentry duty, quite different from my reaction to Bill's non-compliance, which was a patient preparedness for a long, hard haul.)

Changing from active listening to active intervention entailed shifting away from the therapeutic stand in which it was my responsibility to understand the patient's dynamics and interpret them to the patient with judicious timing. I was used to relying on my own training, experience and knowledge, and talking things through informally with colleagues or formally in case conferences. (Often, I and my colleagues would know more about my patients' dynamics than my patients would ever know and, indeed, I believed then it would be inappropriate for my patients to know what I knew.) If my counter-transference became difficult for me, I could take the case into supervision, or I could return for more therapy.

This was in contrast to the approach required by my SCT therapist's role. Not only is the goal for patients to know everything that I know, but to discover it for themselves. In SCT, my responsibility is to orient the patient towards learning how to use the systems-centered techniques and methods so that they can discover their own reality. This requires a focused toughness, leaving the patient no degree of freedom in acting out defenses or the symptoms that defenses generate, and leaving him or her 360 degrees of freedom to make choices as soon as they can contain themselves at the fork in the road and decide which side of the experience they wish to explore first.

This required me to learn skills that I did not have. I was to learn how to be focused and unyielding – to 'keep my eye on the ball' all the time, without taking the excursions into my own free-associations which were characteristic of my psychodynamic self. (This does not mean that I do not have associations to the patients' work in therapy, but they 'just arrive' into my consciousness, rather than being the result of an associative 'search and retrieve.') I was to learn to give up any thought that I knew best about which fork in the road the patient should explore first. This was particularly difficult in that as soon as I thought about the person's dynamics, I was absolutely sure that I knew which was the appropriate choice for the patient to make. Luckily, in the intervening years I have learned, over and over, that, had I influenced the patient to go my way, both of us would have missed something important and something new to the therapeutic system that we were engaged in creating as we worked.

Vectoring

The word 'vector' is used instead of the word 'direction' in talking about the energy of systems because a vector has not only a direction but also a velocity (a driving force) and a point of application (a goal). The concept of vector therefore fits very well with the way that SCT conceptualizes energy. Not only is the word a good way to describe it, but the concept of vector matches both the SCT idea of the fork in the road and also that of the force field which will be discussed later (p.100).

Another important set of vectoring interventions are those that reframe group or individual experience in terms that are depathologizing, legitimizing, humanizing, normalizing and universalizing (one of SCT's goals).

Vectoring interventions make working goals explicit so that the energy of the group-as-a-whole, the subgroups and the members can be redirected towards the work of the group. Vectoring interventions also establish the technique of the 'fork in the road,' which neutralizes ambivalence and conflict by requiring people to choose which side of the conflict within themselves they are going to explore (not explain!) first. The word *requiring* is important here. In SCT, it is the therapist who sets the structure first and then requires the patient to choose how to work within it. Hence the interaction between boundarying and vectoring: the SCT therapist vectors the patient towards the SCT goals using SCT norms. The therapist is responsible for maintaining the boundaries, and for insisting that the patient work within the frame. However, only the patient can test the realities that can be explored within the frame.

The fork in the road

The fork in the road is the technique that implements the SCT assumption that therapeutic change comes when differences in the apparently similar and similarities in the apparently different are discriminated and integrated. One of the strengths of the technique is that it always presents members with a choice as to which of the two aspects of experiences to explore first. For example, in the inpatient unit group, the choice was introduced between exploring an experience and explaining it. By exploring the impulse to explain, members discover that explaining leads them to what they know already, whereas exploring experience leads them to what they don't know. Discovering the unknown is, of course, the goal of therapy. Using the fork in the road technique, members are consistently required to search for, and experience, the active conflict that underlies passive defensive cognitions like ambivalence or cognitive distortions. Discriminating and integrating information is a never-ending process, and using the fork in the road application, we manage regression by integrating the regressive information into consciousness every step of the way.

When members remove their energy from their defenses and vector it to the other side of the fork in the road so that they can explore what they are defending against, they are also weakening the restraining forces and increasing the driving forces.

The challenge to the SCT therapist in vectoring the group's attention is to frame them in such a way that the group will want to turn their energy in the direction that the therapist is pointing. Vectoring interventions re-interpret reality using a different frame from the members' existing map. It is important in SCT that all interpretive interventions are made so that the members can test the therapist's interpretations of reality for themselves. It is for this reason that SCT therapists try to avoid using individual psychodynamic interpretations, but rather frame the dynamic that is relevant to the individual as common to all human beings.

Phases of group development

From the beginning of my group work I had observed group dynamics in the context of the phases of group development as a way of framing the different kinds of work that groups did (and could do) at different times (Bennis and Shepard 1957). It was a revelation to recognize that the different themes around which subgroups spontaneously came together were directly related to the issues that the group had to resolve in order to move from one phase to another in development.

The schema for group development that SCT uses is based on Bennis and Shepard's theory of group development. The phases that they outline trace the development of the group through the phase of authority, in which there is first flight, then fight, culminating in a fulcrum event of scapegoating the leader. The recognition that the issue with authority is displaced from the group's issues with its own authority releases the group from its preoccupation with the leader and enables it to move into the second phase, where issues of intimacy with each other is the developmental task. In the phase of intimacy, the defenses of enchantment and disenchantment against separation and individuation are addressed. When the group has developed a common language that it understands, it has then established a communication pattern that allows the driving forces towards work to be stronger than the defensive restraining force around authority and intimacy. The group has then reached its third phase, appropriately named 'work.'

Just as Bennis and Shepard learned about the phases of development that they presented by observing many groups over time, so I, in my turn, learned about the differences in the manifestation of group dynamics between psychodynamic and systems-centered groups (Agazarian 1994, 1999).

What was common to both of our observational experiences was the sequence of development in groups. Over time as I observed the development of systems-centered groups, I was surprised to note that, although the sequence of the phases of group development remained the same, events that I had taken for granted as inherent to the process of group development were manifestly different. Thus it was not just that the systems-centered approach to leading a group is different from the psychodynamic approach, but that the effect of the SCT approach led to the developmental conflicts manifesting differently. For example, in the flight phase, the SCT group is predominantly compliant but also learning how to reality test. In the fight phase, the SCT group is much more feisty and defiant and exploring the difference between hostility, outrage and anger. In the fulcrum even around their confrontation with authority, the group effectively recognizes the negative transference through the emotional experience of hatred of the therapist. In the SCT groups, through subgroup exploration and the expression of both the hatred and horror, members learn to bring their hatred into their relationships with the therapist and with each other. Shifting into explorations of intimacy with each other, the SCT group changes its character again towards the deeply personal in relationships, and does the work of separating and individuating.

These differences were not only due to functional subgrouping. Modifying the defenses at the boundary consistently weakened the restraining forces and released the inherent driving forces towards development and transformation. For example, in crossing the boundary from the flight to the fight phase, the more passive defenses give way to more active ones. The group that has been through these phases has developed a working containment in which whatever dynamics surface later can be explored and many aspects of development are revisited. This work is done with courage. Members learn that 'emptiness' is restored when the emotion that has been emptied out is restored, and that falling apart is necessary if they are to fall into their undefended selves. The superficial transference based on personal and interpersonal projection is addressed in the first phase of group development, and the dependency transference is addressed in the second phase. In the third phase, it is the pervasive transference that surfaces, and the individuals and the group permanently change in their capacity for consciousness. In the process of developing systems-centered therapy it became clear that it was boundarying that facilitated the shift from the phase that went before to the one that came after.

In SCT, important connections are made between each phase of group development and the modification of the specific defenses that are generic to each phase. This is not a random occurrence, but a treatment plan that systematically reduces the specific restraining forces (defenses) that are characteristically triggered by the underlying dynamics of each phase, which, when reduced, release the innate driving forces to group survival, development and transformation from a simpler to a more complex system.

It was during the late 1980s that I found myself leading groups that I no longer recognized, and those aspects of the group I did recognize manifested in a different way. For example, the budding SCT groups did not, as I expected from my previous leadership experience, volunteer an identified patient as the star of the flight phase. Instead, the group explored in subgroups the two sides of the dependency conflict (that is otherwise acted out by electing an identified patient) and laid down a foundation for developing functional dependency. Nor did the group members target and scapegoat each other in the fight phase. Instead, subgroup exploration enabled members to experience their retaliatory impulses; to experience the twin responses of pleasure and horror at their sadistic revenge fantasies; and to take a step nearer to being able to contain both the strength of the human drive to survive and the compassion about how easily we humans mobilize our sadism instead of our strength. In the inpatient group, only the preliminary work was done, but was well done, and is a good illustration of how firmly the foundations must be laid if a group is to tolerate later challenges.

From this period of trial and error I learned two things. If I maintained the structure of boundarying (making boundaries at all system levels appropriately permeable to information) the group-as-a-whole discovered for itself the underlying individual and group dynamics that I had hitherto believed it was necessary to interpret. The second discovery was that the techniques for interrupting defensive communications both weakened the restraining forces to group development and at the same time released the inherent driving forces towards survival, development and transformation at all system levels.

I experimented with most of these changes in approach in my training groups before I imported them into my therapy groups. Difficult as these intervening months were, the trainees and I learned how to survive the turbulence of the transitions and to discover what occurred when new ways of leading and of exploring came together in a working partnership. We began not knowing where the journey would take us. Often, the edge of the unknown felt like pure chaos to me, and it was all too easy to become afraid that we were creating a monster rather than a group. However, gradually a structure emerged from the chaos. The relationship between interventions and change started to take shape. The SCT hierarchy of defense modification was discovered and formalized. Its major advantage was that the skills, acquired in the process of modifying one defense, simultaneously laid the foundation for acquiring the skills needed to modify the next. The more structured the defense modification skills became, the less chaos erupted in the group. It became clear that defense modifications have a natural order of simpler to more complex, and that this order applies to the phases of development of all systems: member, subgroup and the group-as-a-whole. Thus by modifying the defenses that are generated in one phase or subphase, not only did it become easier to do the work that is important and specific to the particular developmental phase, but it also became easier to make the necessary transitions into the next phase.

Hierarchy of defense modification

With much speculation, experimentation and exploration with training group members, the SCT hierarchy of defense modification was formulated. There were two important outcomes. First, it became clear that the defenses that were generic to the particular phase of development were relatively easy to modify: it was attempting to modify defenses that belonged to a more advanced phase in a less advanced phase that were difficult. Second, it became clear that by modifying defenses in sequence, the skills required for any one modification grew naturally out of the skills acquired before, and laid the groundwork for the skills required next. For example, undoing the anxiety-provoking thoughts made it possible for members to explore the realities that the thoughts were distracting them from. It then became possible for members to explore and undo their tension without the negative predictions that increased it. Undoing tension paved the way for exploring physical experience (like the experience of frustration) without either tensing against it or believing it was too uncomfortable to contain (in fact, it was often the tension in frustration that was uncomfortable, not the frustration itself). These and other discoveries along the way surprised everybody. For example, the difference between anxiety and excitement is sometimes simply the word – and without tension and negative predictions, frustration is often simply an experience of energy and readiness.[5]

The final outcome was a blueprint for the practice of systems-centered group psychotherapy – a guide to the therapist of 'what to do when' in each developmental context – and a treatment plan which predicted that by modifying the restraining forces specific to each phase, the defenses and symptoms that they generate will be modified at the same time. We had, in fact, discovered that there was a natural order to therapy. Restoring the cognitive faculties of reality testing by undoing the anxiety-provoking thoughts that distort reality and generate anxiety was a necessary first step before restoring the connection between the mind and the physical experience of emotion. Restoring the connection between the mind and the body not only made the boundary more permeable between apprehensive and comprehensive experience, but also reduced the tensions and somatic symptoms that occur when energy is misdirected into the body instead of used to understand normal human frustrations and conflicts. Acquiring more frustration tolerance and an increased ability to contain impulses instead of acting them out were the necessary conditions for the next step, which was to make the connection that depression is the retaliatory impulse turned on the self, and sadism is the retaliatory impulse turned on the other. This effectively laid the foundation for undoing depression and exploring sadism and the rest of the hiearchy of defenses (see Table 3.2, p.112) (Agazarian 1997).

The SCT treatment plan

The SCT treatment plan is a sequence of pre-identified phases, each one of which is like a step towards reaching the goals of therapy. It is assumed, in SCT, that there is an inherent drive towards survival, development and transformation in every living human system, defined for group therapy as the systems of member, the subgroup and the group-as-a-whole. It is also assumed that development requires change, and that change means letting go of the known and exploring the unknown. Every human being is both curious and apprehensive at the edge of the unknown.

When curiosity is mobilized as well, apprehension becomes a driving force, opening a door to discovery. Curiosity serves the drive to change. Apprehension, if mistaken for fear and converted into anxiety, generates resistance to change. When the changes confronting the group members as the group develops are not too big, then resistances to the changes are relatively easy to decrease. When the changes are too big, then resistances to change increase. SCT addresses this issue by placing great emphasis on developing a readiness for change before the group and its members enter a new phase of development or before they leave an old phase.

Two sets of criteria assess readiness for change in SCT. The first is whether the group members have learned the SCT techniques for modifying the defenses and symptoms that serve as restraining forces to their own and the group's therapeutic development. The second is whether the SCT skills of subgrouping are established well enough to contain, explore and integrate the conflicts that are inherent to the phase of development that the group is in. If the group dynamics specific to a phase of development are contained, then the group can shift into the next phase without the risk of precipitating an uncontrolled regression.

The outcome criteria for successful SCT work is an increase in emotional intelligence, common sense and humor. This is acquired through developing the capacity to recognize and address the fork in the road between defenses and the conflicts, impulses and emotions that exist in the here-and-now which require containing and managing.

Systems-centered therapy and the inpatient group

SCT expects some turbulence at every boundary crossing. All therapists have to cross the boundaries themselves at the beginning of a group, and depending on what the context is, they will experience more or less turbulence. What is interesting about this fact is that it is the beginning of the group that has such an impact on the process of that particular group meeting. So, in a sense, unlike some other forms of group therapy where the therapist sits and waits for the group to establish itself, the systems-centered therapist has to be prepared to manage both his or her own turbulence at personal boundaries and at the same time manage the boundaries and the boundarying in the group. This was a particular challenge for me as I was beginning the inpatient group, as so much was at stake.

The script in Chapter Two covers the first hour and a half of a brand new group, and from it you should get a good feel for what happens in a beginning SCT group. What you will not get is the way that SCT groups change their character from one phase of development to the next. You will also not have the opportunity of observing how a systems-centered group starts off looking very much like a leader-centered group, and ends up looking very much like a group-as-a-whole group in which the leader is useful only when the group has difficulty undoing a particular defense, has trouble identifying the implicit subgrouping or becomes too apprehensive to take the next step into the unknown.

What you will see is how, from the first few minutes of a systems-centered group, I introduce the SCT vocabulary and the methods which establish the characteristic norms of an SCT group. You will also see how the work with individual members is synchronized with the training steps that need to be established in the group in order to develop the systems-centered norms.[6] Thus the individual who works is chosen by the criteria of relevance to the group development as well as the development of the individual.

Notes

1   The Tavistock model was developed at the Tavistock Institute in England and was based on the work of Wilfred Bion. Tavistock groups interpret to the group-as-a-whole rather than to the members. The equivalent institution in America is the A.K. Rice Institute.

2   In fact, what we have re-discovered is that the lower the functioning of the person, the harder it is for them to discriminate between the work they are doing in their sub-group and the work that the other subgroup is doing, particularly if the 'other' sub-group is exploring envy or spitefulness and so on. This is not a surprise. What is a surprise, however, is that the continuing requirement to contain and to discuss the experience of taking things personally does seem to develop, in the more sensitive people, the ability not to take things 'just' personally, and to discuss, in a subgroup of people who know what it is like, the almost unbearable pain of taking things personally.

3   The most familiar one-up/one-down relationship is any status relationship that has a built-in implication of superior and subordinate. Less familiar are the subtler forms of one-up/one-down relationships that are elicited by posture, tone or attitude.

4   Normalizing is an important technique in SCT which explicitly legitimizes all human dynamics as normal and deliberately refrains or discourages any interpretations that imply they are pathological. The purpose is to legitimize exploration of all human impulses (which then makes it less likely that they will be acted out).

5   Those who are interested in a more in-depth exploration of the relationship between phases of development and SCT should consult the following: Agazarian 1994, 1999, Agazarian and Peters, 1981.

6   As I have discussed, these norms are brought into being by four specific methods that put into practice a theory of living human systems (Agazarian 1997). The group structure is oriented through boundarying interventions; the group process through functional subgrouping interventions; the group goal direction through vectoring interventions; and the establishment of a system hierarchy through contextualizing interventions that develop awareness of how member and subgroup and group-as-a-whole 'systems' have different roles and different goals from the person system (the personal and personalizing experience of the people as they enter into a new group).

CHAPTER TWO

The Verbatim Script of an Inpatient Group Psychotherapy Session Using the Systems-Centered Approach with the Therapist's Reactions

This chapter presents and discusses the full script of a one-time group of patient volunteers from Friends Hospital, Philadelphia, held in 1994. Those who may have wondered how systems-centered therapy (SCT) looks in practice will have the opportunity of following the verbatim script of this hour-and-a-half group session from the beginning to the end. The goal of the group was to see if systems-centered methods applied to an inpatient population would achieve the same results as they do with outpatient and training groups. Seven patients who had been hospitalized for between one and five days and two ex-hospital patients from an outpatient group volunteered to work with me. The session was filmed and a small group of therapists from Friends, other hospitals and private practice came to watch. This was the test. I didn't know whether or not SCT would work for inpatients or, indeed, if it would work at all under the stress conditions that both the patients and I would be working. It turned out, I think, that I was rather more stressed than they were!

I came to the group knowing nothing about the history or diagnosis of the individual patients. I knew only that I would be working with between six and nine members, that there would be both men and women, that some were on medication and some not, and some were new to the hospital and some were not. It was, as you can imagine, a very important moment of containing at the edge of the unknown – not knowing how the group would react to SCT, not knowing how the group would react to the cameras and microphones, not knowing how the group would react to the members of the supervision group who were watching, and not knowing how I would react with so much at stake.

I started the group on time, and after the first few minutes, I found that I was absorbed in the working 'group,' with feelings and experiences not very different from those I'd had with any of the new groups that I had led as demonstrations in front of my colleagues. Looking back, I am grateful for the many opportunities that I have had to demonstrate group therapy 'on stage' and also grateful for the relative absence of self-consciousness that I now experience when I do this. This is not to say, however, that I was not nervous at the beginning of this group. One thing I did notice is that my memory for the details and words of what people were saying in the group was not as sharp as it usually is, and I did not have at the tip of my tongue exact quotes or re-runs of the group process which is a facility that is so useful in SCT. Be that as it may, we all did the best we could.

If this was to be a valid test, it was important that I do the group 'by the book.' So, as you will see, I followed the SCT protocol. We crossed the boundaries from outside (camera and lights and people) to inside and came together around feelings of anxiety, excitement, calm, curiosity, detachment and of being a 'guinea pig.' We undid the anxiety with the *three questions*, roped flights to the past and the future into the *here-and-now*, and introduced *the fork in the road* as a choice between '*sitting at the edge of the unknown* in a new group,' or 'repeating the things you already know how to do.'

The patients were generous, responsive and understanding and helped each other to do what they all agreed was very hard indeed: work in the present. We ended the group (it lasted about 90 minutes in all) with a force field of satisfactions and dissatisfactions (Agazarian 1997). We reframed each satisfaction as a guide to 'what to do more of' in their next therapy group. We framed each dissatisfaction around the disappointment of not doing what one wanted to do, and looked for 'one small thing' that got in the way that they could 'do less of' in their next therapy group (weakening the easiest of the restraining forces). The group ended with encouraging feedback, and then its members left and continued to subgroup outside. I, and all of those who watched it, were moved. To me, it was an awe-full experience of living human systems working together. A great satisfaction was that the process of this experimental group mirrored the process of the experiential training group of hospital staff members that had just preceded it. Thus, it was also a reassuring test of whether or not SCT does what it says it will do and whether it can do it consistently, even when the population and the conditions change.

The patients and I sat in a circle in the center of the room. What follows is a short description of how they seemed to me. To respect their privacy, I have changed their names.

SAM is the first person to my left. Sam is a slight, fair, wiry man with a worried, nervous manner and hesitant speech which he punctuates with many hand gestures. He is in good contact whenever he speaks or is spoken to, has a friendly smile and a good sense of humor.

AL sits between Sam and Bill and is the second person to my left. Adam is a dark haired, solid-looking man, articulate and insightful about his own obsessive defenses. He sometimes responds to the group with curiosity and interest and his full attention, and at other times appears withdrawn, preoccupied or depressed. He is probably on medication.

BILL sits between Al and Josh, the third person to my left. Bill is a heavy-set man with a large belly and an air of authority. He has clear and well rationalized opinions which he uses to make his case. He is given to story-telling as a defense and is able to be both oppositional and co-operative.

JOSH sits between Bill and Nan, and almost opposite to me. Josh gives the impression of a keen intelligence with which he is observing the group and the leader. He seems both intensely curious and puzzled by the process. He wears a yamaka and has his hair in a pony tail. Josh seems unlikely to accept anything until it makes sense to him. Unfortunately, he does not appear to have access to his emotional intelligence, and so he is at a loss when he is asked to pay attention to the here-and-now.

NAN sits between Josh and June and is also almost opposite to me. Nan gives the impression of a plump child who is anxious to please. She sits sprawled back in her chair, her legs off the ground, and lets the group go by. She does not initiate things in the group, but can respond and become engaged when the therapist helps her to focus. Her major defense is the 'oft-told tale' which has a flavor of being honed in therapy. Her feelings are close to the surface and she probably 'floods' easily. It is also probable that in her understanding, flooding with feeling is therapeutic.

JUNE sits between Nan and Pam and is the fourth person to my right. June responds slowly in the group and tends not to initiate. She appears comfortable, content and somewhat unfocused. She looks sleepy. Her mood is probably influenced by medication. June fully believes that her current peaceful sense of well-being has come from learning how to love herself.

PAM sits between June and Jane, the third person to my right. Pam came late to the group because she had an appointment with her psychiatrist. She is an alert, smallish woman who appears to be 'with it' in the group. She does not initiate much, but follows the group process with full attention and is clear about her opinions about the process.

JANE sits between Pam and Rose, the second person to my right. Jane is a slight woman who is at times quite vague and non-committal, and at other times focused and clear. Her body language ranges from passive, helpless and quietly oppositional to active and co-operative. When she is not hiding herself in a smoke-screen of vague language, she can stand up for herself and her opinions which are often different from mine.

ROSE sits next to Jane on my immediate right. Rose is an attractive, slim woman who appears self-possessed, sure of herself and skeptical. She varies between being somewhat aloof and oppositional to being involved and spontaneous. She is highly articulate and aware of what is going on in the group. She has moments when she is either briefly depressed or preoccupied.

ROSE   YA [the author]

JANE

SAM

PAM

AL

JUNE

BILL

NAN

JOSH

What follows is as close as possible to the verbatim script of the work that these patients did in the group with each other and with me.

Beginning the group

I am already sitting in the circle when the patients come in and take their chairs. The room is large, and the chairs are grouped in the middle, surrounded by cameras, microphones and lights. In the corner, across the room from the door, is a group of observers from an ongoing SCT Supervision Group. When the patients have settled themselves, I begin, looking around the group as I talk and making eye contact with some of the members.

> YA: Okay. Well, first of all, I want to thank you very much indeed for being part of this. This is the first time that I have worked inside a hospital with this method, so in a sense we are all pioneering. So I want to thank you very much for volunteering.

In my first words to this beginning group I am introducing the context: the reality that this is an experimental group that we are all taking part in. This is the first step in recognizing a common experience, which is the basis for the SCT method of functional subgrouping.

Functional subgrouping

A systems-centered group is brought into existence through subgrouping, which brings members together around similarities. You will see below how I elicit similarities around the common theme of the members' experience of being in this group. Before, however, encouraging verbal subgrouping, I first set the stage for nonverbal subgrouping by making sure that all members can see each other. Encouraging members to look at each other as they talk encourages them to pay attention, both to what they are saying and to the other members of their subgroup. Maintaining eye contact and joining with a similarity rather than separating with a difference are the two basic principles that establish functional subgrouping. SCT leaders establish functional subgrouping in the first few minutes of a new group which establish norms of communication within the group that are identifiably different from other beginning groups.

> YA: And the first step is to make sure that everybody can see everybody. So, can everybody see everybody without any difficulty? Not the people out there (*referring to the group of observers*) – we will deal with them in a minute.

By moving my chair as I talk, I am modeling, and indeed, some of the patients move their chairs (although, as they did not look around to see if it was necessary, it was a move that had more to do with 'follow the leader' than it did with its purpose!). This small moment of behavior has two important implications. First, the group is co-operative – it is not going to sit there immobile in passive resistance. Second, it is compliant to the leader.

It goes without saying that it is not functional for a group to remain fixated in compliance to the leader. However, in a beginning SCT group, compliance is functional in that it makes it easier for the SCT leader to introduce and establish the norms of behavior that are essential if the group is going to develop the norms that make an SCT group.

As the members move their chairs, Jane, who is next to an empty chair, points to it and looks to me. I respond:

> YA: We have – I think someone will be joining us later – I don't know if… (*The group tells me she is with her doctor.*) Okay, she is with her doctor at the moment.

Boundaries: Separating outside from inside

> YA: So the first thing is, how is it for you, in here, on stage, with me, and with people watching, in front of the camera? How is that?

My question acknowledges the context, and also asks the members to take the first step in joining the leader and the group: 'How is it for you, in here, with me?' In these first few moments I am intending to set the stage by acknowledging the context, in reality. Legitimizing reality reduces ambiguity, and reducing ambiguity tends to reduce the anxiety.

It is an input that is intended to make the reality of the world 'outside' the group explicit so that the work of crossing the boundary from outside to inside could begin. The reality is that this group of nine people (eight present, one to come) is sitting in the middle of a room in a circle, surrounded by cameras and the camera crew, with the hospital supervision group sitting in the corner, members of whom, throughout the first ten minutes of the group, came in late.

'Telling it like it is' is fundamental to every systems-centered group in that it is the first step towards living in the present. In SCT, we call this 'crossing the boundaries into the here-and-now.' In SCT, boundaries are understood to be imaginary lines in space and time. Space boundaries mark the threshold between inside the group and outside the group, not only in the real space that the chairs define, but also the psychological space that is defined by which way group members direct their attention. It makes a big difference to how much energy is available for work if the members can keep their attention focused on the work of the group. Boundaries in time also exist both in the real world of clock time and in the timeless psychological world of the past, present and future.

What I have failed to do, responding to my own stress, is to tell the group what the real time boundaries are: what the exact stopping time for the group is, and how long we have to work. Setting time boundaries at the beginning of a group is one of the ways that SCT establishes group structure (which I typically emphasize to supervisees). By failing to structure the time boundaries I leave unnecessary ambiguity in the group.[1]

What happens next in the group is a live example of how defenses in a group emerge in a natural sequence, nested inside the phases of group development. From repeated observation of the sequence the *Hierarchy of Defense Modification* was developed (see Table 3.2, p112). Anxiety is the first defense to be modified in SCT; the thoughts that generate anxiety and anxiety-provoking thoughts are the defenses that are most likely to inhibit a beginning group.

> YA: So the first thing is, how is it for you, in here, on stage, with me, and with people watching, in front of the camera? How is that?
>
> Group: Nervous! (*says one member*) Nervous (*echoes another*).
>
> YA: Nervous. (*Reflecting and legitimizing the members' words.*)
>
> Rose: Doesn't bother me!
>
> YA: It doesn't bother you at all. Okay.

You will note how small bits of speech are cues as to whether the speaker is attuned to the person to whom they are responding. My adding 'at all' was a failure in attunement with Rose.

> Group: Exciting (*says a fourth*).
> YA: Doesn't bother you – and – exciting. (*I am acknowledging the last two members.*) So we have two 'nervous,' one 'exciting'...
> Bill: Doesn't bother me.
> YA: So you are in the same boat with Rose.

I am introducing the SCT functional subgrouping 'boat' language and am joining the two members together with a look and a gesture.

Functional subgrouping is the major factor in developing a systems-centered group. It is also the major challenge to members as it requires joining members around similarities rather than staying safely individualized in differences. This requires members to communicate in new ways, which is a challenge to the comfortably familiar.

> Bill: I was on live TV...
> YA: So you've got some bigger things. (*I laugh nervously.*)

With the adjective 'bigger,' I am aware of another attunement failure. (It is doubtless no accident that Bill and Rose were to become the subgroup that contained the group resistance!) I guessed that Bill was about to use the familiar defense of 'story-telling' and I was trying to interrupt him before story-telling became established in the group.[2] Working from a negative prediction like mine does in fact take one out of attunement with the other and into attunement with oneself.

Introducing functional subgrouping

> YA: So now we have got two 'nervous,' one 'exciting,' two 'not bothered.' Anyone else?
> Sam: One 'guinea pig' (*shrugging and throwing up his hands*).
> YA: One 'guinea pig' (*with a responsive laugh*).

I am attempting to establish a low-stress climate by continuing with supportive reflections, and – in the case of the complex joke 'guinea pig' – lightening the atmosphere with a laugh rather than focusing on the underlying implications.

> YA: One 'guinea pig' and... (*looking around*)
> Al: Curious!
> YA: Curious.

Subjectively, I am astonished and delighted, both by the responsiveness of the group and by how the responses spontaneously fulfill the basic SCT criteria of entering the unknown with curiosity. The group is responding with feelings and experience, not intellectualizing, explaining or explaining away, and bringing in diversity and curiosity. No SCT therapist could wish for more.

The groundwork for subgrouping has now been built, and I introduce the first of the SCT defense modification techniques.

Undoing anxiety

Technically, the first defenses that SCT modifies in a group are social communication and defenses against anxiety, tension and irritability, in that order (Agazarian 1997). In this group so far, there is little social behavior (with the exception, perhaps, of the story-telling 'defense' of Bill). As the communication in the group is relatively non-defensive (the energy is so far available for subgrouping), the first task for the group is to modify anxiety in an 'anxiety subgroup.' Modification of anxiety is done by getting members to 'discover the reality' that feelings come from two different sources: anxiety comes from anxiety-provoking thoughts, and from misinterpreting the physiological signals of emotion (panic attacks, for example, escalate if the person becomes anxious about their heart rate and breathlessness). The third source of anxiety is a misinterpretation of the natural apprehension that occurs in uncertainty – which can change into excitement and arousal if curiosity about what comes next is aroused.

The 'three questions for anxiety' are:

1. Are you thinking something that is frightening you? If so, then the member is asked to identify the anxiety-provoking thought which is frequently a negative prediction or a fear of what others are thinking.

2. Do you have sensations or feelings that are frightening you? If so, then the member is asked to describe the physical sensations and to make room for them. In the process, it is usual for members to recognize that the discomfort arose from their attempt to constrict their emotional experience, and when they relax, their experience changes to a pleasant sense of energy. Sometimes the major difference between anxiety and excitement is the word we call it!

3. Are you sitting at the edge of the unknown and feeling anxious about it? If the source of anxiety is the third question, then common reality is affirmed with 'everyone is apprehensive at the edge of the unknown and it helps if you can take your curiosity with you.'

> YA: We have a lot of different things to work with in the group. I want to start, if I may, with 'nervous' – because, very important in this

method is knowing where one's anxieties come from. And sometimes they come from one's thoughts and sometimes they come from one's experience. So for – who – who was – ah, you were nervous? (To June.)

June: Being here.

YA: Okay – and who else was nervous? (*Nan and Rose gesture.*) Okay, and you (*to Sam*) were nervous and a guinea pig! Okay (*Sam and I laugh together*). In terms of being nervous, do you four (*gesturing to them*) know whether you were thinking about something that's scaring you?

June: Never being in a group with lights all around me and people behind me listening to what's going on – other than in a small group of people with the same problems.

I am introducing the beginning of defense modification into the group. However, as it is a beginning group, the first step is to subgroup again, so that the first member to begin to work with their anxiety will be less likely to become an identified patient and more likely to be one of a working subgroup. So, when June says 'never being in a group with lights all around me and people behind me listening to what's going on – other than in a small group of people with the same problems,' I respond immediately, and introduce systems-centered concepts and vocabulary.

Curiosity at the edge of the unknown

YA: Yes, so you are right at the edge of the unknown in a sense.

June: Mmm.

YA: You are right in the new experience?

June: Right.

YA: Okay. Do you have any thoughts that make that experience any worse – or is it just that it is new?

I am checking to see if the anxiety is the expected apprehension of being at the edge of the unknown or whether June has anxiety-provoking thoughts that are contributing to it.

June: It's new and I'm curious!

June has put together for herself 'curiosity at the edge of the unknown.' I am again grateful for the spontaneous contribution, by a member, of one of the important principles of SCT. There is always some apprehension at the edge of the unknown, and the apprehensive experience changes when curiosity is mobilized, probably because it shifts the focus from anticipatory anxiety, which is a restraining force, to interest, which is a driving force. I reinforce the idea that apprehension at the edge of the unknown is normal and mobilizing curiosity reduces it. I smile and say:

> YA: Okay! All right. Well what I find is if I go into something new and I am a little anxious, being curious is really helpful.
>
> June: Mmm.

The SCT rule of thumb is to refrain from any self-disclosure in the first phase of the group. The exceptions to the rule are the generalizing interventions that SCT therapists make with the intention of normalizing human experience. These interventions are designed to create a climate in which all aspects of human experience can be explored without fear of being labeled by the self or the other.[3] In this context, therefore, the therapist's self-disclosure reinforces the idea of the shared humanity of everyone in the group.

> YA: So you are in a good place for being here. (*I then return to subgrouping.*)
>
> YA: How about you two?
>
> Sam: This stay here is the first time I had any kind of therapy and I am not too familiar even with therapy I'm in as it is, and I am a little nervous about being here, but I figure, anything that can help…it's worth giving it a try…

I am intensely involved in what he is saying – we already have some connection over the guinea pig joke. He looks distressed and is not altogether easy to hear; however, he is making good eye contact. I have a slight uneasiness that this group is his first therapy experience since admission, and am relieved when he says 'you know, it's worth giving it a try.'

> YA: So you are also on 'the edge of the unknown,'
>
> Sam: Yeah.
>
> YA: And curious? (*reinforcing the connection between being at the edge of the unknown and curious*) – and you are sort of hoping it's going to be good!
>
> Sam: Yeah.
>
> YA: Okay. So you've got two realities and one wish.
>
> Sam: You've got it! (*His tone lightens, and he half smiles.*)
>
> YA: Okay (*I smile back*).

Separating reality from unreality

With this intervention, I am introducing a discrimination between the world of facts and the world of ideas. Consistently encouraging members to make discriminations is fundamental to SCT therapy, and is based on the assumption that living human systems survive, develop and transform through the process of discriminating and integrating differences. If this is in fact true, then increasing the ability to discriminate differences in the apparently similar and similarities in the apparently different will be the only dynamic that it will be necessary to influence. Functional subgrouping is the method that puts this idea into practice.

Next I turn to Jane, the last member of the nervous subgroup.

> YA: How about you? Are you thinking anything that is scaring you?
>
> Jane: No, uh, I don't know, haven't given it that much, you know, real thought about it.

Discriminating + integrating differences

Ambiguity defense

Jane is obscuring, one of the ambiguity defenses. Obscuring is a particularly frustrating defense in that it is like a smokescreen which makes it difficult to make contact with the person who is hiding in it.

There is a heavy emphasis in the practice of SCT on reducing ambiguities, contradictions and redundancies in communication which act like 'noise' in the communication process and make it more likely that information will get lost. Obscuring and other forms of ambiguity not only interfere with the relationship with others, but also with the self. This is particularly important in that SCT assumes that the prerequisite for therapy is a real relationship with the self, which then makes it possible to have a real relationship with another. It is also assumed that a real relationship with the self is a prerequisite for work in therapy.

As Jane is saying that she has not given it much thought, she is sitting passively, with her hands hanging loose on the arms of her chair. Flaccid hands are a signal that the person is not involved in what she is saying.[4] I am therefore not going to put pressure on Jane until there is more support for exploring resistance.[5] I do, however, want to see if she can connect with her subgroup. So I say:

> YA: And is it also for you that it is right on the edge of the unknown?
>
> Jane: Yeah, I guess. (*Jane's voice is expressionless. She shrugs. Then suddenly, with quite a bit of energy, she says:*) Of course!

This sudden infusion of energy into her hands and her voice is an encouraging signal and allows me to believe that we might do some work later. For now, I draw her attention to a discrimination.

YA: So you have just shifted from guess to certainty? (*Jane nods and I return to promoting functional subgrouping.*)

YA: So we have three people who are a little bit anxious about not quite knowing what's going to happen next. Has anybody else joined these three? (*Looking around to see if there is unacknowledged membership in the group.*) Anyone else joined since we've been working?

I'm redefining the subgroup and checking to see if anyone else is working along.

Al: Yeah, the more I have been sitting here the more I have become curious and also nervous, instead of just curious. More might be going on but I am still curious about it.

YA: Yes.

Al: I'm still a little nervous about what might be going on, but I am still curious about it.

YA: Yes, and you don't have any thoughts that are scaring you?

Al: Not at about this situation, no!

I am wondering if he is making an allusion to conflict outside this situation, so my next comment reinforces both boundarying and subgrouping.

YA: Okay, so as long as you keep your attention in here you've got lots of company, about being a little anxious (*Al nods and he says 'right'*), not knowing what's going to happen (*'right'*), and also curious (*'right'*). It's a great way to start as we are open to whatever happens then.

Addressing the silent subgroup

I then look around the group and ask 'How about you three?', addressing the three members who have not yet spoken. Josh answers. He is aware and focused, and gives the impression of an intelligent man, puzzled by the process.

YA: How about you three?

Josh: Physically I am a little tense, or becoming tense. I am not quite sure why, exactly.

Tension in the silent subgroup

Josh has spontaneously introduced into the group 'tension,' the next defense that is modified in SCT. This is based on the observation that as anxiety lowers in a group, tension rises. I take advantage of this to introduce the SCT hypothesis of 'tension as a straitjacket that constricts the experience of emotion.' At the same time I reinforce reality testing in the group by asking the member to check it out with himself – in other words, to become a researcher of his experience…

> YA: One of the ways that we think about tension is that we sort of clamp down on our body and stop ourselves from having feelings. Now, that is not necessarily what is happening, but is it possible that the tension you feel is stopping you from feeling something?
>
> Josh: Well I am not sure. I don't feel like I have, er, anything at stake.

Josh is intellectualizing, and probably unaware that there is a difference between thinking and feeling. Substituting the words 'I feel' for 'I think' is a common intellectualizing defense in therapy.

> Josh: So there is sort of, uh, no reason that's visible to me why I should be tense…
>
> YA: Uh huh. So you are…
>
> Josh: …but physically I am a little tense.

'Turning on' the researcher (see p.34, endnote 6)

> YA: Are you curious about why you are tense?

With this intervention, I ignore the temptation to modify his intellectualization defense and continue to promote subgrouping around curiosity.

> Josh: Yeah, actually I am.
>
> YA: Okay. So we don't know at the moment. It may be that you are having a feeling that you don't know about.
>
> Josh: Maybe.
>
> YA: Or it may be something else. We will just have to wait and see.

Here, I am continuing to emphasize the reality testing approach to 'discovering reality,' which is one of the major orientations of SCT.

> Josh: Maybe, uh, I have had the same feeling before both in situations where I was consciously nervous and sometimes in situations like this one where I don't see any reason that I can attach why I should be nervous.

Discriminating between inter-system and intra-system experience

> YA: So in a sense your unknown is what is going on inside you. We have a sort of subgroup here where the unknown is not knowing what

> is going to happen here (*referring to the edge of the unknown subgroup*).

(*Group: Murmur of assent.*)

YA: And in a sense, your unknown (*looking at Josh*) is you don't know what is happening inside you. Is that right?

Josh: I guess so.

YA: You guess, or, this *is* what is happening?

This intervention is again targeted towards modifying ambiguity. This seems particularly important with Josh, who is showing a tendency to ruminate about reality rather than to experience it. When his response is tepid, you will see that I reframe it in terms of 'waiting to see' (sitting at the edge of the unknown, not knowing).

> Josh: Well, I am not sure, so I'll accept that interpretation at the moment.

YA: Okay, so we'll have to wait and see?

Josh: Sure.

YA: Okay. How about you two? (*Looking to the silent subgroup.*)

Bill: Well, as I said before, in 1982 I was on the *People are Talking* show with Maury Povitch. I belonged to an organization called Parents without Partners...

YA: If I may interrupt you?

Bill: Sure!

YA: How about right here-and-now?

Modifying social behavior: The story-telling defense

This is the SCT technique of immediately interrupting a characteristic 'social' story-telling defense before it becomes entrenched. The interruption serves two purposes. The purpose with the member is to bring him back into the here-and-now and encourage him to notice how he is managing himself in the present. It is also a training intervention for the group, reinforcing the focus on the here-and-now. The intervention attempts to modify two boundaries of the story-telling defense: the first from inside to outside and the second from the present to the past.

In SCT, keeping people connected to both the here-and-now of the group and their conscious, present selves are the primary goals of the first phase of group development.[6]

> YA: How about right here-and-now?

Bill: This second?

YA: Right. How are you right now?

Bill: Relaxed.

YA: You are relaxed. Are you comfortable?

Bill: Fine. I just wiped out the fact there's...I know there's a camera here and I know there's people over there, but I'm oblivious to it.

YA: So you've done something to wipe it out? (*I am wondering about Bill's defenses. Does he ignore stressors in the here-and-now, and does that leave him relaxed?*)

Bill: Yes.

YA: And then by wiping it out you are relaxed?

Bill: I think it's because I did have the experience. The first time I was on TV I was nervous. But because I've had the experience before – er – when it first started and when I was on the program, I was nervous for a while but then I forgot the audience was there and the cameras were there and I was interacting myself. And I...

YA: ...mmmm?

Bill: ...and I had no idea that we were going to have this today, the cameras.

In SCT, we as therapists prefer to encourage the members to explore and discover their dynamics from their own experience rather than interpret them to them. The disadvantage of interpreting (as I did to Bill above) is that I, not he, made the connection between relaxing and wiping out the stressors. My interpretation was built on a hypothesis about Bill's defense pattern. His first line of defense is the social defense: he 'tells stories.' When he is in interaction, he explains. By ignoring reality he maintains and reinforces the cognitive map which explains reality to him. By explaining he does not explore, and by not exploring he does not discover whether or not his map is an accurate or an inaccurate picture of the here-and-now. He relaxes when he ignores reality, but at the cost of being out of touch with reality. If he does not discover this for himself, it is unlikely he will change his map. I attempt to lay the foundation.

YA: So, right now...

Bill: I am still relaxed.

YA: So, *right now!* So right now, you ignore the cameras...

Bill: And the people...

YA: And the people...and you are relaxed here?

Bill: Mmm.

YA: So how are you, being in the group with us? Do you have a feeling about that? (*Attempting to connect Bill to the here-and-now.*)

Bill: A feeling about that? I am just wondering how I am going to react when we start interacting with each other.

YA: Just hold it a second – you just went off into the future! (*Immediate boundary work – from the future back to the present.*) You see, you just wondered about what's going to happen. How about what is happening right this moment? (*I keep connected to Bill.*) Do you have any experience right this moment? (*pause*) In the present?

The third member of the silent subgroup

I look around the group slowly, and back again to Bill. I have put out an alternative framework and wait to see if he is able to work within it. He does not seem to have a reaction (his map leaves him few degrees of freedom) so I turn back to the group again with 'anybody else?'

Bill has been the first member who is warding off my SCT influencing attempts – so far. I wonder if he is the spokesman for non-compliance. At the very beginning, he had came out of left field and I half-fumbled the ball. In this last interchange we approached reality from two different directions. Josh, who also approached reality from a different direction, joined me in a willingness to test an SCT hypothesis, but there is no response from Bill. This feels to me that it may be a moment of transition, where the differentiation between a 'co-operative, compliant subgroup' might become differentiated from an 'uncooperative non-compliant subgroup.'

YA: Anybody else?
Nan: Scared.

Nan 'looks' like a compliant member. Her posture is almost childlike. She is heavy, and sits as if she has no bones. Her voice tone gives an impression being both eager and pleased to respond. In this sense, her words (scared) don't match the sound (pleasure).

YA: Scared, okay. How about you? (*I turn to Rose.*)

Nan has made a bid to work on fear. However, Rose is the member who has not yet joined the group with any feelings, so before we go deeper in the group with Nan, I want to see if Rose can join in the subgrouping.

Rose: I am just here (*there is no expression on Rose's face*).
YA: Okay. No feeling yet?
Rose: There's nothing to have a feeling of.

YA: There's nothing to have a feeling of.

Rose: Because I don't know what is going to happen, so how can I make a judgment about it? I am just waiting to see.

In contrast to Bill, Rose's affect is flat. My internal feeling is that this may well be the transition into the non-compliant subgroup. What is more, my heart drops a little when she implies (as Bill did) that she is 'waiting for something to happen' – which is so different from my own experience in which so much is happening.

Failed subgrouping

YA: So in a sense you two are somewhat in the same place. You are both waiting to have a feeling about something that is going to happen in the future?

As I say this to Rose, I gesture between her and Bill, connecting her with Bill to see if she will subgroup. Rose smiles at Bill, and is blank of face again when she looks back at me. I feel reassured that she does have interpersonal affect but is in a role-lock (SCT language for the early transference relationships) with me and/or my role.

Rose: I don't know if I would term it that I am waiting to have a feeling. (*Rose is definitively joining the subgroup that is going to hold its own ground against me, and I feel it!*)

YA: Okay.

Rose: I am just...

YA: How would you term it?

When I ask Rose 'How would you term it' I am using the SCT discipline of transferring the locus of change from me to her, and giving leadership over to the group in the person of Rose who is implicitly subgrouping around the role of resistance with Bill. In the back of my mind I have the impression that there is a co-operative subgroup that is following my lead and a non-cooperative subgroup that is maintaining the group potential for testing its reality and testing its leadership.

Rose: I am just... (*Rose goes through a transition at this point. Her face is still immobile while she says this. Then she pauses, considers what I asked her and turns to look at me.*) How do I feel right now? Is that the question? (*As she asks her question we make contact, and a small eruption of laughter breaks through her impassivity.*)

YA: Mmm.

> Rose: I just feel… (*Her tone is changed and while she is considering, I cue her.*)
>
> YA: Right in the present!
>
> Rose: Okay, I'm relaxed.
>
> YA: You are relaxed. Okay. Is that comfortable?
>
> Rose: Yes. (*She and I smile at each other.*)
>
> YA: Okay. All right.

For me, the tension is reduced and I am relieved that we have made a contact. There has been a reversal from a defiant to a compliant role relationship to me. Was the incipient struggle between Rose and me bypassed for the moment when I asked her 'How would you term it?'?

Compliance in the beginning phase of a group serves as a driving rather than a restraining force in that it makes it possible for the members to learn a significant amount of the methods and techniques which will later open the door to their being able to manage their defenses themselves. In SCT there is always the hope that they will learn enough of the techniques to help them explore their defiance when they shift into the fight stage rather than act it out.

The silent subgroup has clearly been carrying the resistance to the SCT process. Bill is not committing himself but is also not story-telling. Josh has compromised and agreed to test a hypothesis. Rose has shifted into compliance. In a sense, the social behavior is now in the service of co-operation – a restraining force is now a driving force.

At this point I resume the work of undoing anxiety in the group and turn back to 'scared' Nan.

> YA: And you're scared?

Now that all members are subgrouped, there is a group-as-a-whole safety net for Nan who looks as if her affect may be more labile than the others (and is therefore a potential candidate for the identified patient). At this point, two things happen in the group. First, the missing member, Pam, comes up to the group and pulls out her chair. I say 'Hello' to her. Before I can turn to Nan again, Bill takes up the gauntlet – 'May I ask you a question?' As you will see, this struggle for control of the process is more overt (general and outside the group viz. specific and here-and-now). But whereas a tentative alliance was forged between me and Rose (tentative in that Rose stays related to Bill with head nodding), there is no rapprochement between me and Bill. Rather, there is a brief skirmish which I win. In the therapist's chair with the power and influence that carries, it is no surprise that I win.

Managing a challenge to SCT here-and-now norms

Bill: May I ask you a question?

YA: Yes.

Bill: We are all in different stages of being in the hospital ...

YA: Well, we are all in the same stage of being in this new group.

Bill: I am talking about being in the hospital.

YA: Uh, I am talking about being in the group (*an overt power struggle*).

Bill: Okay.

YA: Would that be okay if we stayed and focused on the group?

Bill: Yeah, that's fine. The only one thing I wanted to say though, is the fact that if this had been a week ago, and you had asked her that, she might have said 'I'm scared' because she was in a different situation a week ago. Today, you see, she's got the medication under control, she is fine. I am still, you know... I just came in on Saturday, so like I said, we are all in different stages of medication...

YA: Right.

Bill: And...maybe, you know, later on (*gesturing to Nan*) she wouldn't be scared.

Late member

YA: Right (*I say, turning away from Bill and directing attention towards the new member*). And we also have a brand new member who has only just come into our group.

This is one of the moments in SCT when maintaining the SCT frame competes with attunement to a resistant member. Had this been an ongoing group I would have responded to the situation by asking for a subgroup, so that other members would be able to subgroup with Bill and explore the issues involved in focusing on the past or the future rather than the present experience in the group. This would be the preferred response in that it would both give Bill a subgroup to work in and at the same time give the group an opportunity to explore a different position to mine.

There is also the issue that the absent member has just joined the group and if she is to be able to work in the group, a bridge between her and the group will have to be built. As you will see, in giving her a summary of the process and purpose of the group so far, the new member gets some orientation to the work that has been missed. At this I look to the group for validation, to see if what I thought I was doing checked with what the group experienced.[7]

YA: ...and we also have a brand new member who has only just come into our group.

Pam: Yes, who apologizes for being late, but her doctor held her up.

YA: Yes, okay, and I want to thank you for volunteering. I have already thanked the group, and we have done, er, some work, and the work that we have done so far is that we have just begun to separate out the experience that comes from our thoughts (*I look away from Pam, around the group and back again*) and the experience that comes from our feelings – and we are also just beginning to separate out things that come from thinking about the future and what it is like to have our experience in the here-and-now. (*I look around the group again.*) Does anyone recognize that that's what we've been doing? (*There is a murmur of assents in the group.*) Yeah, okay, how is that? My thought is that if we pay attention to the here-and-now and learn how to manage our experience with each other, *right this moment*, we have got a good chance of learning how to manage things on the outside. If we use this moment to learn what is difficult for us, or easy for us, we will also learn about managing outside. (*There is a lot of focused attention in the group.*) Where we are right this moment is (*letting the new member know that we had been working with Nan by turning to Nan*)...

YA: (*To Nan*) You said you were scared? I am going to ask you the same question, which is: are you thinking something that is frightening you?

This is the first of the three questions which are intended to help Nan identify the source of her anxiety.

Nan: Yes.

YA: What are you thinking?

Nan: Oh boy! I am really scared now.

Nan's reaction continues to be discrepant in that she is smiling and looking delighted, while at the same time claiming that now she is really scared. The SCT response, at this early stage in the group, is to educate. The contradiction between the words and the feeling would not be addressed in an SCT group until members had acquired the ability to be curious about their own discrepant reactions rather than to feel put on the spot.

YA: Well, you know, thoughts that are inside one's head...

Nan: Mmm... (*She nods like an obedient child.*)

YA: …are always more frightening before you put them into words. So will you say what your thought is?

Nan: Okay, that's true (*Nan continues to be compliant*).

YA: So, would you test that out?

Ideally, the goals of all SCT interventions are framed as hypotheses that patients can check by exploring their own experience. In SCT language, this is the source of experiential or apprehensive validity.

Nan: Okay, I will. (*She takes a deep breath and looks up to the ceiling.*)

In SCT work it is assumed, when people's eyes look up towards the ceiling before they talk, that they are likely to be thinking, most probably as a defense against connecting to their immediate experience. Thus, they are likely to be taking the fork in the road towards 'explaining' their reality rather than 'discovering' it through exploring their experience in the here-and-now and seeing if it is the same or different from their explanations. SCT encourages a constant awareness of the fork in the road between defenses (like explaining or explaining away experience) and the reality of experience. This is also called 'keeping people in a box' – a box in which the only exit is into the self.

Keeping Nan 'in the box'

Nan: I have a way of covering up my feelings with my family…

Nan begins to 'tell her tale,' the reciting of which appears to give her great satisfaction. It is probable that Nan's interpretation of herself has been developed and polished in previous therapies, so that she now presents it as an explanation for her difficulties. These explanations rarely enable patients to make the changes that they have come to therapy to achieve. As you will see, following the SCT guidelines, I will encourage Nan to pay attention to the facts of her experience rather than her oft-told tale. I interrupt her:

YA: Okay. Right this moment, you said you were scared.

Nan: Yeah. It's, it's, let me just… (*holds up a finger as a way of influencing me to let her make space for herself. I ignore the finger and I continue to redirect her focus away from 'explaining herself' towards 'exploring her experience.'*)

YA: Is there anything at all that you are thinking…?

Nan: Yeah (*her finger goes up again – again I ignore her signal*).

YA: …about this group?

Nan: Yes (*finger goes up*).

YA: What?

Nan: Just a few minutes ago (*she holds her finger up high as if pointing*)...

YA: Yes?

Nan: Just a few minutes ago I went outside and met my dad.

YA: Uh-huh. (*I say this with some caution, not knowing whether this is fantasy, hallucination or reality.*)

Nan: And it frightened me.

This is one of those moments in the group when a lot is happening at once and I had to make some judgment calls. For my own comfort, I wanted to assess whether Nan was hallucinating.[8] From her manner in the group so far, it was possible.

YA: Okay. So you went outside and you *thought* about your dad?

Nan: I thought about him and I got all upset, and my stomach started turning. (*Nan's hands go round and round, illustrating how her stomach turned.*)

YA: Was that while you were in this group? (*Orienting question about space and time.*)

Nan: It was right before I came to this group.

YA: How about since you've been in this group? Has anything happened?

Nan: I feel more calmer.

YA: You do?

Nan: Mmm.

YA: So is there anything that is frightening you right now?

Nan: Uh. (*This time Nan stays in eye contact, appears calm and appears to be checking with herself.*)

YA: Do you feel frightened right now?

Nan: No! (*She shakes her head with assurance. She is no longer showing any signs of agitation.*)

This is the second time that I have kept a patient in the box with the intention of restoring the connection with the non-defensive self. In the first, with Bill, I 'won' (as at this stage of the group, what therapist wouldn't?) and Bill had been compliant enough to allow himself to be redirected (but there were not yet good enough signs that he could actually make use of the redirection). With Nan, however, keeping her 'in the box' resulted in her becoming able to notice her experience in present reality and potentially contrast it with the unreality that she built with her thoughts.

Contextualizing: Working for the group as well as the self

> YA: Okay. So, you see, what you have just done for us is to show us that we can leave the group and go outside to thoughts that make us very uncomfortable. But when we match those thoughts with what is happening in the group, we feel better.

I am using the same frame that has been used earlier, the difference between discomfort that is generated by thoughts with which people leave the group, in contrast to the direct experience of the moment. I am also reinforcing the connection between the individual member and the group, and emphasizing that the member's work is for the group as well as for him or herself. At the same time I am reinforcing the connections between what is being demonstrated in the work of the group and the principles that can be learned from it.

> Nan: Mmm.

> YA: So we come from the outside into the inside and sometimes it is hard to stay right here. (*I am acknowledging the reality that continuing to cross boundaries in order to stay in the here-and-now is in reality a difficult task, and asking if members are experiencing the difficulty.*) Is anybody finding it difficult just to stay solidly in the group in the here-and-now? (*Al signals with his hand and other members nod. This response is satisfying evidence that the group members are working along with each other.*)

> Al: Yes, I am.

> YA: Yes (*to Al – and then, gesturing across the group to the other members*), yes – we have others? (*Several members murmur their assent.*)

Work

> YA: Yes…you have…you have…yeah (*acknowledging the potential subgroup*).

> Al: As long as things are fairly static I tend, my mind tends to go towards, er, other worries and concerns about other aspects of my life.

> YA: Right.

> Al: And then as soon as something starts happening in the group, uh, then I sort of (*gestures with left hand*) like put that down for a moment. I check out what is happening (*gestures with his right hand*).

> YA: Yes.

> Al: And if it interests me I stay with it, if not, I go back to whatever, uh, things I was worrying about. These would fall under mostly

work-a-day worries – job, apartment, what am I going to do in a couple of weeks...

YA: So let me...

Al: ...this friend, that friend...

YA: So let me interrupt you and bring you back into the group. So if you stay in the group, you don't worry?

Al: (*Pause*) Right.

By SCT criteria, Al is available to 'work.' His 'observing system'[9] is mobilized in that he can clearly describe the way he divides his attention between his worries and reality. Potentially, therefore, he has access to both kinds of experience: the experience that is generated by his anxiety-provoking worries and the curiosity that gets him to 'check out' his environment.[10] With this clear discrimination, he can be introduced to the idea of choice. This is in contrast to the earlier work with Bill, who 'wipes out' his experience in the present by escaping to his narratives about the past or speculations about the future. Bill is not yet able to work as he is distracted from his real experience not only by his defenses, but also by the defiant and compliant roles he takes in relationship to the therapist.

The initial work in SCT is to mobilize a system that is able to observe the fork in the road between the defensive roles and symptoms on the one hand and the direct personal experience that is being defended against on the other. As soon as this is recognized, the patient can begin the work of exercising choice.

Choice – Preceding fork in the road work

YA: Okay, if you had a completely free choice, which would you rather do – stay in the group or go out and worry?

I frame the conflict in terms of the 'fork in the road' and introduce the idea of choice – to relate to the reality of group or to relate to his worries.

Al: (*Answers immediately*) Stay in the group!

YA: All right, so you have a sort of goal for now – learning how to stay here. (*I relate the choice to working towards a goal.*)

We exchange a smile. With this interchange I have the kind of experience therapists get when we 'bond' with a patient, and in fact we have established a working connection that persists until the end of group. I feel the pull to continue working with him, but to do so would be at the expense of the group and would run the risk of volunteering him as an identified patient. So I rely on subgrouping to connect him to the other members of the group.

Al: Yeah.

YA: Yeah, and you have a companion over there. (*I relate the work to a subgroup, connecting Al with Josh. Then to Josh I say:*) You were also noticing you were having difficulty...

Josh: Yeah...

YA: ...staying in the group. Is that the same kind of thing, or different?

Josh: Well, essentially I've been searching my memory to see if I can remember when I felt the exact way before and see if it's different.

YA: You mean tense and not quite certain why?

Josh: Right, and how that compares to other more disturbing anxieties.

YA: Okay, so what I'd like to say to you also, if you go outside and back into your past and match what's happening now with what's happened before, you may come up with a good explanation, but what you would miss is anything new you discover from living in the here-and-now. So if you can stay... (*pause*) being tense is not all that comfortable is it?

This contrasts two ways of gathering information: the fork in the road between crossing the boundary into the past, and trying to explain the present from the past on the one hand, and on the other hand, discovering the experience of the present by staying in the here-and-now.

Josh: No, actually I'm somewhat less tense now.

Josh is manifesting an ability to be aware of his physical experience – the question is whether he can also become aware of his emotional experience.

YA: Good. Still a little tense? (*Reinforcing the reduction in tension – checking the reality of 'somewhat' tense.*)

Josh: Yep.

YA: So if you pay attention to your tension *here* there may be something that happens that you don't know – if you just sort of explore the experience and wait and work in the group you may just discover that there is something that you didn't know about yourself. And certainly what we're here to do (*I look around the group again*) is to learn some things about ourselves that we don't already know – because we all already know how we get into trouble.

YA: (*To Bill*) Have we lost you? What's happening with you?

I had experienced a failed connection with Bill in the previous interaction, about which I was uneasy. However, it turned out that he has been 'working along' with Al.

One of the major advantages of the group is that it enables members to work vicariously as another member does work that they themselves are not ready to initiate. Bill has been silently resonating with Al (the original member of this subgroup, now made up of Al, Bill and Josh).

Work and spontaneous subgrouping

> Bill: I agree with you, I think I just sort of feel it the same as you do (*points to Al, but stays looking at me*) as far as if I have my mind occupied. It is like a façade (*he draws the invisible façade in front of him with his hand*) and I'm hiding my feelings inside too.

Bill is thoughtful as he speaks. The incipient rebellion is over. There seems to be a co-operative working climate in the whole group.

> YA: Yes? (*I'm moved.*)
>
> Bill: I mean it's like, you know, whenever I feel like I'm on stage – going on stage. (*He makes his façade gesture again.*) It's like I can work on my problems later, after this is over with. (*Al glances at Bill a couple of times while he talks.*)
>
> YA: Uh-huh.
>
> Bill: …get it done first, and worry about my problems later on.
>
> YA: Uh-huh, so it is not altogether real for you right now?
>
> Bill: Uh, no.
>
> YA: Okay, is anyone else feeling like that? (*I glance at Al.*) You just smiled if you noticed. Is that because you went off outside or has that something to do with this?
>
> Al: Both. Both, they're the same thing.
>
> YA: Same thing?
>
> Al: I tend to – uh – I have – uh – one way of reaching my sense of identity, which is how much I can worry, how much I have to worry. For some reason, it seems to be one way that I identify myself to myself.
>
> YA: Yes.
>
> Al: There are other ways that don't involve worry but it is the most debilitating.
>
> YA: Yes, if we just stay with that for a moment. You have got one way of feeling like yourself, which is by worrying? (*Al nods*) Okay. Well the issue for all of us here (*looking around the group*) is finding out ways that you can feel like yourselves when you are actually

living in the here-and-now. And you know, the here-and-now for us is in this group and being together. Does anyone have a sense for how you can feel like yourself right now? We are beginning to learn a lot about things that pull us away; (*to Nan*) your thoughts about your father before you came to the group; (*to Al*) your worries that give you a sense of yourself but stop you from being here; (*to Bill*) your worries; (*to Josh*) some of your tension. So what are some of the other things that stop us from being right here?[11]

Rose: By not focusing on being here now?

YA: Yes.

Rose: By considering the past and the future instead of the present.

YA: Right. (*To Bill*) The same with you?

Bill: Yes!

Rose: It is not – uh – it is a matter of focus. (*The interchange with Rose supports my message, but I did not feel the resonance.*)

YA: Yes, so in a sense you have a struggle to focus on the here-and-now. Do you get pulled away into the past and the future?

Rose: Everybody does.

YA: That's true.

Rose: I think that's normal to have that happen, but I have been working on that a lot because in my company we have this saying, 'be here now.'

YA: Yes.

Rose: So it is something that I have been working on for over a year and I find that the more I do it, the easier it becomes.

YA: So, as you practice that right now, how is your experience?

Rose: I am able to stay here.

YA: Yes.

Rose: Most of the time.

YA: Okay, one thing I am wondering is, if we look at each other more whether that helps us stay more here, if we sort of look around the group.

Eye contact and a break in the video-tape

One of the major reinforcers of SCT group process is the consistent emphasis on eye contact. The group had done sufficient preliminary work in resonance and it seemed as if the members might be ready to increase their contact with each other.

However, there was always the risk that they were not ready, and that too much intimacy, too soon, might jeopardize the climate which was beginning to feel very good. I was therefore reluctant to introduce this next step. I was also aware, as the group made eye contact, that I was only working with this group for this one time, and that the patients themselves came from different units and would not be continuing together. I wondered what the effect of 'meeting' each other's eyes would be, and whether it would arouse feelings that would not be sufficiently contained in the group and that would result in depression.

It was a moment of great conflict for me. If I was to test whether SCT would be appropriate for hospitalized patients, I wanted, as much as possible, to lead this group 'by the book.' My emphasis on the importance of eye contact, my question as to whether early misatunements could be modified through the different stages of eye contact in subgrouping, and the concern of some of my therapist friends that eye contact could not be tolerated by hospital patients made it extremely important not to let my anxieties influence me.

It was a very uncomfortable moment, and it was very ironic that the section which contained whatever information there was to be seen in this section was lost in the changing of the tapes.

During the period that the tape was being changed, the members of the group looked at each other round the group, making and maintaining eye contact in silence for a length of time that surprised me. They seemed interested as they made contact, and occasionally smiled at each other. The supervision group recalled it as an intensely moving moment which seemed important both to them and to the patients.

Certainly, the level of emotion deepened in the group when the video started up again. Bill is talking, telling the group how much therapy he had, but how he had never cried in therapy – that he always cried alone.

Bill: If I can't cry...I mean, same thing – no way – you ain't seen me cry.

This is a tender issue for everyone in the group. Bill was now introducing an issue that relates to his relationship with himself. By SCT criteria, it could be a big step forward for him. I was unsure, however. He may simply be introducing his next 'symptom' (his inability to cry with anyone).

If I had been doing 'individual therapy in the context of the group' I might have been tempted to encourage Bill to cry. From the SCT frame it is important not to push any one member into the depths of his feelings without a subgroup. With a subgroup, members go no deeper than the subgroup can go. This is frustrating sometimes for members who are ready to go further. However, it also builds a 'floor' in the group so that the group-as-a-whole steadily increases the capacity to experience emotion without its members flooding or regressing. SCT labels a sudden regression into flooding emotion a 'deep sea dive' and explicitly discourages it by saying something like 'before you go too deep, let's see if there is a subgroup, so that you do not have to explore these feelings alone.' This offers an alternative to one of the familiar events in group therapy, where one member will have a storm of emotion while the other members watch. Managing emotion in the group in this manner is often said to be cathartic for the patient, and good for the group. Through SCT eyes, however, the patient who volunteers for the 'catharsis' is likely to have had it many times before and therefore suffers both the pain and pleasure of repetition.

So, instead of encouraging Bill, I interrupted him and checked out whether Bill is a 'voice for the group-as-a-whole' and whether there is a potential subgroup to work with him. The two members either side of him were looking down.

YA: Hold on a moment, we just lost two people. Was there something about what... (*To Bill: 'What is your name?'*)

Bill: Bill.

YA: Is there something about what Bill said right then, about having feelings in private but not being able to have them with people, that sent you off?

Al: Yeah.

YA: And is there anyone else also who's...

Rose: Yeah.

YA: Yeah, okay. Anybody not in that group?

Group: No!

Josh: I'm not.

At first, it looks as if the group-as-a-whole is ready to explore feelings. However, very soon it is clear that there is another round of defenses to modify before deeper interpersonal relationships can be addressed.

YA: You're not. You can have your feelings with people also?

Josh: Oh! No! Well, I wasn't reacting particularly to what Bill said.

YA: Okay.

Josh: You saw me looking at the floor?

YA: Right. Do you know what you were reacting to?

Josh: Uh, well, basically to you. I am trying, er, to figure out that, what you are trying to do so that I can, er, see whether or how I, er, I can get some value from it.

YA: Do you have any question you'd like to ask me?

I am hearing Josh as a voice for the subgroup that wants to know more about where I am leading before going there. His is an important statement, in that he is taking a neutral rather than a defiant or compliant stand. His statement is an opportunity to harness his intelligence to the work of preparing him and the group before taking the next step.[12] When differences with the therapist are expressed openly in the group as a serious query, it lays the foundation for reality testing in the group. Thus SCT thinks of this as the loyal opposition.

Loyal opposition

> Josh: Uh, well, I have one objection, which is that I don't buy at all, that, uh, the way we, er, learn new things about ourselves or anything is by, uh, uh, excluding, uh, the past and the future, uh, I think there is very little completely experience-free learning for anyone, uh, uh, old enough to remember anything.

> YA: Okay, well, I wouldn't argue with you. I wouldn't disagree. What I would say though, is, if in this group today what you do is, er, *think explanations*, what you won't have the opportunity to do is to explore your experience right in the moment.

> Josh: Well, I figure, that's why I am trying to figure out what you are doing and where you are going.

> YA: Okay, so do you have...so I wouldn't disagree with you, but do you see that you are at a fork in the road? One fork is: you are wondering what I am doing...

> Josh: Mmm...

> YA: ...and the other fork, which you are apparently not paying attention to right now, is exploring your experience while I am doing it.

> Josh: I am trying to see that fork, it is not easy to see at all.

> YA: Right, but I don't think you can do it both at once, you know.[13]

> Josh: Maybe not.

> YA: Yeah, I think you can, uh, okay, I think that if you could wonder later and just pay attention to yourself right now – would you be willing to try that?

> Josh: Well, I am trying to do that, it's...

> YA: ...right...

> Josh: it's very, very hard to...

> YA: ...yes...

> Josh: ...engage...

> YA: ...right...

Josh: ...your full attention on the present...

YA: ...absolutely...

Josh: ...unless the present itself is providing an enormous amount of...

YA: ...right, absolutely...

Josh: ...stimulation.

YA: And in our present here, we were just, I think, on the threshold of beginning to explore what it is like not being able to bring our feelings out into the present. Is that what we were beginning to explore? Is that good competition for you incidentally? (*Looking at Al*) Your concern about your worries that they take you away but at the same time they give you a sense of yourself?

Al: Yeah, it's a...

YA: ...do your feelings also give you a sense of your self?

Al: Yeah, but they're not always, er, they're not always pleasant and yet they...

YA: So right this moment, do you have a feeling?

Al: Er, yeah.

YA: Okay. Is it pleasant or unpleasant?

Al: Sort of unpleasant (*half smile – possibly anxiety*).

YA: (*I smile back*) Sort of unpleasant. Okay, so what is it that's happening right now, do you know, that's giving you an unpleasant feeling?

Ambivalence

Al: I – I think we are all just playing games. I mean, we are all, we are all ambivalent.

YA: Yes.

Al: Or mostly...

YA: Yes, so let me say something about...

Al: I don't like being, you know, I don't like thinking about being at a fork in the road, or...

YA: Okay, yes.

Al: ...or, or having a feeling but not being able to let them out, or not having a feeling... (*Al's hands are gesturing from one side to the other, on the one hand this, on the other hand that, and his voice is sounding frustrated – a graphic communication of the anguish of obsessing.*)

YA: Yes, sure.

Al: It's all new and this bothers me a little bit.

YA: Yes.

Al: It isn't actually – and sort of extra different view…

The last three members have deepened the work in the group, acknowledging that change is not easy. From the SCT frame, ambivalence is a cognitive defense which avoids the experience of the underlying conflict. The SCT approach requires undoing the ambivalence defense by drawing the ambivalent person's attention to the passivity and lack of involvement in the underlying conflict that ambivalence avoids. Once the conflict is engaged, the person has available two experiences pulling in different directions, and therefore a fork in the road and an available choice as to which side of the conflict to explore first. It is interesting that the word ambivalence means 'two' and 'valence' – two forces of different valences, vectored in different directions!

> YA: Yes, well, let me say something about ambivalence. Ambivalence is a way of not struggling with conflict. See, ambivalence lives in your head. The conflict lives in your experience and, I agree with you, I think right now trying to bring ourselves in and have some kind of meaningful experience with each other is not easy and I think it does confront us with our problems.

This is the SCT 'teaching' that ambivalence is avoidance of conflict – again acknowledging the reality that the work is not easy and does confront members with their problems.

> Al: Yeah, the reason I am here is because I don't handle conflict, that kind of conflict resolution very well. (*Al gives an anxious half-laugh.*)

Here Al spontaneously relates his ambivalence to conflict avoidance which leads to the SCT requirement to reframe ambivalence as a fork in the road so that the patient can choose which side to explore first.[14]

> YA: Okay, well…excuse me… (*I've interrupted, but Al gives a 'be my guest' gesture*) …how do you think you are handling it right now?

> Al: Er, er, er, I am just sort of going along with it. I don't want to…uh…I don't want to make any type of commitment to any particular, er, er, point of view right now.

There is an opportunity here to join Al and Josh in a subgroup. Instead, I continue to work with Al attempting to make the fork in the road operational.

> YA: Right.

> Al: Er.

YA: Right, sort of sitting on the fence?

Al: Er... (*Half nods and then shrugs.*)

YA: No?

Al: Er...

YA: Or more in than out. Or more out than in?

Al: Sitting on the fence and not wanting to make a commitment to...er...put my chips down in any particular spot...whatever.

I now reframe 'sitting on the fence' as a positive action, one in which Al can explore the choice about whether he wants to take himself further in, or further out of group. It's important to notice that there is no value judgment. All that matters, in SCT therapy, is that the members learn to discriminate and integrate in an interpersonal climate of authenticity. Thus as long as members are paying attention to choices and learning from exploring both directions, work is being done that, according to the theory, will promote system development.[15]

YA: Yeah, but you know, sitting on the fence is a very good place to be, to look down both forks in the road. When you are sitting on the fence like that, you begin to have a choice about whether you want to take yourself further out of the group (*looking around the group*) or whether you want to bring yourself further into the group.

I am now looking for resonance and subgrouping. The group members are attentive and participating. There is a group interaction and a group joke about the fence – and later, some demurrals.

Spontaneous subgrouping around work

Al: Sure...

YA: Yeah. If you can stay present! Anyone else sitting on the fence like that?

Jane: Uh, I think I do.

YA: (*Looking back at Al and joking*) But you have to hang in on the fence! (*Group laughter.*)

Rose: (*To Al, joking*) ...because if you don't you're going to fall in off the side.

Bill: You can become enamored of the fence too.

YA: What?

Bill: You can become enamored of the fence too.

> YA: That's true, that's true, that's when you go back up to your thoughts.
> If you actually keep yourself on that fence and ask yourself every
> second, which way do you want to go — do you want to come
> into the group, meet people, do some of the work of learning
> how to share feelings? Or do you want to go back to the ways
> that you know already — how to defend oneself — which we are
> all very good at.

While I am talking, Bill is wiping his eyes with his hand. Sadly I do not see this until I am watching the video-tape, and therefore do not have the opportunity to acknowledge that he has tears in his eyes.

> Bill: I'd like to share my feelings, but, man, I don't know how to.
> YA: Okay.
> Bill: But I'd like to.

I suggest action for Bill, an interaction with the group by making eye contact, which may connect him to people in the present and perhaps give him a fork in the road between his experience relating to his thoughts about himself and his feelings, and an experience of being himself that he will be able to compare against his thoughts. This would be a first step in revising his cognitive map.

> YA: Well, a first step might be to look around the group and see if
> anyone else wants to share their feelings also. We don't know
> how to do it, we haven't done it yet in this group.

This is also an important technical moment. The group members are getting closer to relating to each other. Bill is developing a salience for leading the group to the next step. He has come in with a clear statement of wanting to share his feelings. The fork in the road for me is between working with him directly and reducing the restraining forces that are preventing him, or connecting him to the group in a subgroup that is trying to learn how to do the same thing. The choice for me here, where the group is still in the early phases of formation, is to continue to encourage the group to take each new step together, reducing the restraining forces with any members who may be left behind. Josh, Nan, June, Pam and Jane have had very little interaction so far, although from the nonverbal responses they appear getting ready to join.

It is important to note how easily and unwittingly a therapist can influence the communication pattern. It is true that most of the interaction has come from the side of the group to my left, and it is also true that I have reinforced the interaction to my left. I am aware at this point that it would be important to support interaction from the other side of the group. However, notice that I am subject to the dynamics of group just as the members are, and it takes some time before the communication pattern shifts.

> YA: (*Reprise*) Well, a first step might be to look around the group and see if anyone else wants to share their feelings also. We don't know how to do it, we haven't done it yet in this group.
>
> Sam: I'm on the fence.
>
> YA: You're on the fence with him. (*I connect Sam and Al with a hand gesture.*)
>
> Sam: I am leaning toward jumping in.
>
> YA: Okay. (*I smile and we connect.*)
>
> Sam: But let's...
>
> Bill: I have a problem with the fact that when I am upset with something I'll tell somebody else about it and let them do the dirty work.
>
> YA: Uh-huh.
>
> Bill: I don't...I'm not a very combative person.
>
> YA: So do you know who you would like to have do your dirty work in here?
>
> Bill: I haven't decided yet! (*General laughter and supportive reactions towards Bill.*)
>
> Bill: I haven't decided. (*The group continues to enjoy the joke.*)

This, from a SCT point of view, is a good example of how laughter can be either a driving force or a restraining force depending upon the context. Currently there is solidarity in the group, and an ability to work together and support each other as preliminary to subgrouping. This is a context in which laughter is a driving force. This laughter is not a defense against working, but part of the climate of work.

One of the characteristics of this group that has been reassuring is the congruence between the gestures that members make and what they are saying. Now, there is an additional spontaneity in the laughter, and freedom to laugh and joke with each other.

Spontaneous contextualizing

> Josh: No, I'm just not experiencing it that way. I'm trying to be both self-aware and sort of fully engaged in what's happening in here.
>
> YA: Right.
>
> Bill: So far I haven't managed to get my mind around that. I've been working on that.
>
> YA: But it seems to me that that's very important for all of us (*I make revolving eye contact around the group as I talk*) – how we can both

pay attention to each other and the group and also pay attention to ourselves. It seems to me that that's a very important experience, which in a sense we are all working with...

Once again there is a lot of focused attention from the group on what I am saying. I am introducing the last step of the interpersonal interaction.

SCT understands three different levels of system in group: the member, the subgroup and the group-as-a-whole. It is when these three systems are communicating that there is maximum potential for the people who are in the group to get therapy. However, before these three levels of systems can manifest in the group, the people who join the group have to 'learn' how to become systems-centered members, which is what most of the work has been about so far.

In order to become systems-centered members, people have to leave their outside roles outside and join the group with their energy in the here-and-now and learn how to take on the systems-centered role. The first step in becoming systems-centered is to recognize that their relationship to themselves has two parts to it: a thinking part and a feeling part. This then allows them to relate to themselves in two ways – a thinking way and a feeling way – and to learn the difference between the fork in the road that leads to explaining and the other fork which leads to exploring, which is so essential to systems-centered work. The group is already working well 'discovering reality.' The group had started with two subgroups on this: one that was focused on the unknowns in their relationship to the group (their environment), and the other focused on their unknowns in relationship to themselves. The members are consistently paying more attention to themselves and beginning to report what they know about themselves in the here-and-now. The next step is to have them pay attention to themselves and also to another. When we talk systems we say it is the intra-system and inter-system: when we talk people, we say intrapersonal and interpersonal.

> YA: (*Looks at Al*) You're sitting on the fence partly paying attention to yourself outside the group and partly paying attention to yourself inside the group – is that right?
>
> Al: (*Nods.*)
>
> YA: Still doing that?
>
> Al: (*Nods, we maintain contact and nod together.*)
>
> YA: Okay. (*To the group:*) So, we are sort of at a fork in the road. Can we bring ourselves more in with each other talking about things that have some meaning to us in relationship to what is going on now?

Dependency question

> Pam: I'd say as a member of previous groups…I have had a lot of group therapy before so I know the struggle of the here-and-now and dealing with the rest of the things later. That is what individual counseling is for, so I would say that for me, being part of this group, even though I came in late, I already feel like I am in the group, but I didn't know exactly what issue it was that you wanted us to talk about.

This is a good illustration of the contrast between the group-as-a-whole discipline and SCT. In group-as-a-whole work, Pam is representing two things for the group. One is membership, both as the late member, and also as a member of the silent subgroup in the group. The second is the bid for the leader to lead – to tell the group what to do. In my group-as-a-whole role, I would not respond with an answer giving an instruction. I would put the issue of what to do back into the group, either with an intervention (preferably a group intervention) or with silence.

In my systems-centered role, however, three things are of importance. First, the silent subgroup is getting a voice. Second, the member who has in reality missed some of the orientation work is asking for direction. Third, and most important of all, the context of Pam's question is at the beginning of a new 'education' phase in a group that is mainly working in functional dependency.[16]

Goal-oriented answer

> YA: Well, the issue that I am wanting us to talk about is learning more about what stops us from being who we want to be when we are anywhere. And at the moment, where we are is this group. So what do we know about what stops us from being who we want to be in this group?

I pause, staying connected to the silent subgroup on my right. The response, however, comes from Bill, who is one of the members of the active subgroup. There is an interesting group dynamic issue at this moment. Groups learn fast from reinforcement, either explicit or implicit. The active subgroup in the group has mostly been to my left (with the exception of Rose who is sitting next to me). Therefore there has been more interaction between me, the group and the active subgroup – who are also all men. Thus there has been an implicit group reinforcement to interact more with one half of the group than the other. As we are now at the boundary between individual work and group-as-a-whole exploration into what stops people from being who they want to be in their world, it is important for me to reinforce the participation of the silent subgroup. At the same time, I do not want to disturb any of the work that is emerging spontaneously.

This transition point, the transition between work that is predominantly weakening the restraining forces at the boundary (defense modification) and more active subgrouping, is always a turbulent one for me – being led by the flow of the group rather than leading it either one way or the other. One nice thing about SCT work, thanks to the fork in the road between defense modification on the one hand and education on the other, is that there is always something useful to do in the group, whichever direction the group takes.

Turbulence at the boundary: Shame

> Bill: I know what stops me, I am sort of ashamed that things are happening to me and don't want to discuss it, you know.
>
> YA: Right in this group you are ashamed of what is happening to you?
>
> Bill: In any kind of group.
>
> YA: So...
>
> Bill: Sometimes even my therapy...
>
> YA: Excuse me, what you have already told us is that it is very hard for you to have your feelings when you are in therapy.
>
> Bill: Mmm.
>
> YA: Okay.
>
> Bill: It is very easy when I am by myself.
>
> YA: Yes, and you are also now telling us that one of the things that stops you is feeling ashamed.
>
> Bill: Yeah, embarrassed, ashamed.

This is a very important threshold. One way of thinking about shame and shyness, embarrassment and feelings of humiliation, are as turbulence at the boundary between the true self and the defended, socialized self. This then becomes a choice between paying attention to how painful the shame or shyness is on the one hand, and paying attention to the motivating want on the other. The *want* is the driving force and the shame or shyness is the restraining force to 'showing' one's spontaneous self.

> YA: You see, I do just want to say something about that. Whenever we bring ourselves in, it is always a little embarrassing, we are always a little bit shy, sometimes we are a little bit ashamed, sometimes we are a lot. But if we pay attention to the embarrassment and the shame and the shyness, we won't be able to bring ourselves in. If we pay attention more to the wish to bring ourselves in, we

have got a better chance. So you are at another fork in the road, if you pay attention to your shame, it is going to be harder for you to bring yourself in *now*.

Bill: The only way I'll know if I've conquered this group is if the tears start running down my face.

YA: Would it be a relief if you did that?

Bill: I don't think so, no.

YA: Okay, you have just made a negative prediction.

Bill: That's true.

YA: How are you doing? (*I ask Al*) Are you still on the fence or did you leave?

Al: Uh, no, still on the fence.

YA: That's great. (*Looking around the group.*) So what do we know about what stops us from being here-and-now in the way that we want to be?

The group is silent but attentive for ten seconds. I am paying more attention to the 'silent' subgroup and am looking to my right. It is, however, Sam, the silent member on my left, who breaks the silence. At this point I am concerned that the communication pattern is already set and it may not be possible to change the activity level between left and right – a negative prediction.

Sam: This fear of opening up in front of a lot of people, it's normal.

YA: We're not saying it is not normal.

Sam: It's...

YA: We are saying, do you want that to stop you?

Sam: No (*emphatically*), I don't want it to stop me.

YA: Well, okay, so do you have a sense for what part of yourself you'd like to bring in?

Here again is the SCT emphasis of bringing the conflict into the context of the here-and-now and seeing what one learns when experiencing the conflict, live, in context, instead of talking 'about' it.

Dependency question

Sam: What do you want to hear from me? Why I'm, why I'm here at all?

YA: Well, okay, so now we have got another fork in the road (*I look around the group again*) – if you're going to bring yourselves in, are you going to bring in the self that I want you to bring in or are

> you going to bring in the self that you want to bring in? Which one would you rather do?

Sam: I want to hear what we are supposed to be doing. I have a million problems outside of here and a million things happened in the past…I want to hear what your program is here and see if it can help.

YA: Okay (*I look around the group again, careful to include the 'silent' subgroup*), anybody else in that boat?

Jane: I'm, I'm with him, I think he made a good point. (*Jane is sitting passively, head submissive, hands folded in her lap, and speaking softly.*)

YA: Mmm, and how would you put it if you made your own point?

I am keeping connected to both Jane and Sam. I am encouraging subgrouping nonverbally, by looking from one to the other. We are still at a very important transition – this time from passive to active. I have made several bids for members to make an active connection between what they want and the way they relate in the group. Bill is at the fork in the road between bringing in the feelings that he wants to bring in on the one hand, and the shame on the other. Sam is at the fork in the road between pleasing me or pleasing himself. Now Jane is at the fork in the road between supporting someone else's point and making her own. Jane is also expressing the loyal opposition of the more silent subgroup.

Jane: Well, uh, I think that, uh, we all are here for a purpose and we all seem to have, uh, barriers we have to get over and, uh (*shrugs*), we should all try to co-operate and, uh (*unfolds her hands and puts them on the arms of her chair and sits up straighter and straightens her head*), you know, and come forth and say what we are really thinking instead of beating around the bush. (*Drops her head and gives me a straight look from under her eyebrows.*)

Jane looks as if she is now available for work. She appears to be connected to herself in the way that was just glimpsed at the beginning of the group, when she responded with 'Yeah, I guess,' shrugged, and then suddenly, with quite a bit of energy, changed from passive to active with an emphatic 'Of course.'

Work

YA: Okay, so do you have something?

Jane: We are all on the fence, let's face it (*sits forward, speaking more emphatically, gesturing with her hands*).

YA: Right.

Jane: We are all on the fence.

YA: Yes.

Jane: So, er, he tried to get off just now by telling you how he felt (*her gestures are larger and more fluid, and she makes a brief fist at 'how he felt.' This is an example of what SCT calls intention movement, which communicates nonverbally an emotion of which the person may or may not be aware.*).

YA: Okay. And you, right this moment?

Jane: And now I do too. (*She still gestures, but now her right hand ends up limp at the end of what she says.*)

YA: Okay.

Jane: So I think I deserve some credit for that (*limp hand again*).

YA: And do you have a feeling that goes along with your thoughts because you're, you're telling us...

Jane: Well, uh, I, uh...

YA: ...what you think? Do you have a feeling that goes along with that?

Jane: (*Jane gives a half-laugh, and blows out with a short breath.*) I don't know, maybe anxiety, I don't know, I'm not sure, embarrassment too (*puts her hands together and links her left fingers into her right*), anxiety, and, uh, a little anger and, and, uh, I don't know, a lot of things.

I am careful to do reinforcement work here, legitimizing anger as another of the feelings that we are 'containing' in the group. Containing in this sense means recognizing a feeling experience and exploring it, rather than acting it out.

Anger and discrimination: Anger as different from the target

YA: Okay, so what you are bringing in that's new for us in the group – because we have had anxiety, we have had embarrassment.

Jane: Mmm.

YA: We have had curiosity and excitement and various other things (*looking round the group*) – but you are also bringing a little anger in.

Jane: Yeah.

YA: Okay, has anyone else got some of it?

(*Silence*)

Sam: I've got some anger at myself.

YA: Let's separate out...

Sam: Okay.

YA: Let's separate out the experience of the feeling of anger and how you target it.

Sam: Mmm.

YA: Because one can have anger and one can target it in all sorts of different ways, one can target it at oneself, one can target it at me, one can target it at the world. But what about the feeling of anger? Have you got a feeling of anger?

Sam: Right now? No!

YA: No? Not yet. (*My voice sounds slightly regretful.*) Okay. Well, that's not going to get you into that boat then. Does anyone have a feeling of anger or do we only have one member? (*Looks around the group.*) No feeling of anger?

Bill: If you had spoken to me three days ago I would have thought I had a feeling of anger. (*Flight into the past.*)

YA: (*Looks at Bill and then at Josh.*) I think we have got some anger right now. Have you got a feeling?

Josh: Yeah, at you.

YA: Okay.

Josh: I still can't figure out what the program is.

YA: Okay, so are you feeling in resonance with the anger over there? (*To Jane*) Did you miss it?

Jane: Are you talking to me?

YA: Yes.

Jane: No.

YA: Did you miss it?

Jane: I, er...

YA: Where did you go? You just had someone...

Jane: Well...

YA: ...a companion in your anger. Did you miss it?

Jane: I think he agrees but I mean, I'm not sure if he really feels anger, I mean...

YA: Okay.

Jane: I don't see it on him. He doesn't look angry.

YA: So do you want to ask him?

Jane: I see other people do but I mean...

YA: So, so who else do you think might be angry?

Jane: Well, a lot of the women sitting here seem to be angry. (*Looks at June.*)

YA: So would you ask her?

Jane: I don't know, ask them what?

YA: Well you just...

Jane: What should I ask?

YA: Go slowly now!

Jane: ...I don't know. (*Laughs*)

YA: Go very slowly. This is, this is...

Jane: I mean, er, I feel that she has, she is harboring some anger.

Checking out a mind-read

YA: Just hold on a second.

Jane: Okay.

YA: You just made an assumption.

Jane: Yeah.

YA: Okay?

Jane: Assuming.

YA: Yes, you made two assumptions.

Jane: Okay.

YA: Okay, you made one assumption that he wasn't angry...

Jane: Right.

YA: ...and you made another assumption that she was.

Jane: Yes.

YA: Okay, now would you be willing to check out your assumptions?

Jane: And what, I wouldn't know how.

YA: Well you could ask a question that would get a yes or no answer.

Jane: Okay, I'll ask, I'll ask a direct question. (*To June*) Are you angry?

June: Not in this group, no.

Jane: Not with anybody here?

June: No, I'm relaxed.

Jane: Just relaxed?

June: In fact I'm getting too relaxed.

Jane: Your demeanor is entirely different to me. (*Laughs*)

YA: (*To Jane*) Just hold on a minute.

June: I could go to sleep, I could go to sleep. It is so relaxing.

YA: (*To June*) So right this moment what you are doing... (*looking to Jane*) What is your name?

Jane: Jane.

YA: (*To June*) You are helping Jane to check her reality, and what you are doing is you are telling Jane that the way she thinks and the way you are, are two different things.

June: Yes.

YA: You are doing some pretty important work. (*To Jane*) Do you believe her, Jane? That (*to June*) – what is your name?

June: June.

YA: So you don't believe that June isn't angry right now, even though she has told you that she isn't?

Jane: Right.

Checking for cognitive dissonance

YA: So how is that for you – to check your reality and find out that June has a different reality from yours?

Jane: Mmm.

YA: ...and you don't believe her.

Jane: Mmm.

YA: How does that feel?

Jane: Well, I feel as though, uh, you know that I have to rethink, but, uh, at the same time my first, uh, my first impression, uh, you know, already said yes...

YA: So it is hard to change your mind, is it?

Jane: Well, not at the moment.

YA: Yes. Is that one of the difficulties you have?

Jane: Yeah.

YA: Okay, so now we have for you, in this group, one of the same kinds of difficulties that you have outside?

The repetition, in a group, where it can be explored and understood with a different outcome, is one of the major powers of group therapy. In an SCT group, the mechanisms for identifying and changing the basic human defenses are a major part of subgroup work, where individual members become increasingly aware that their difficulties are human and that if they are willing to do the work of checking reality, they can undo them as many times as necessary. SCT members are told that it does not matter if a defense re-occurs as long as they are able to notice it, to take their energy gently away from the defense and explore for what conflict or impulse of emotion that they are defending against.

Jane: Mmm.

YA: Okay?

Jane: I guess so.

YA: You guess so or it is true?

Jane: Well, I'll have to say it is true. I totally agree.

YA: Okay, would you be willing to check your reality again now? You had a sense that – (*to Josh*) what is your name?

Josh: My name is Josh.

YA: (*To Jane*) You had a sense that Josh wasn't angry?

Jane: Mmm.

Checking out a second mind-read

YA: Would you be willing to ask him a question so he could say yes or no?

Jane: Well, I could ask him the same question, uh, you, er, mentioned being, feeling angry, uh, were you, are you angry?

Josh: Uh, I don't feel angry right now, uh, I, I think it was, er, pretty much discharged immediately, so I would say that by the time you made that observation, that I would agree with you.

Jane: You would agree with me?

Josh: Yeah.

Jane: Okay.

Josh: By, by the time you made that observation I would have agreed with it.

Jane: Mmm.

YA: So how is that? You've had one who disagrees with you and one, Josh, who did agree. How does that feel?

Jane: So it is not completely, er, false (*Laughs*) on my part.

YA: Well, wait, how is that for you?

Jane: What do you mean?

YA: You were accurate one time and you weren't accurate the other time.

Jane: Mmm.

YA: How is that for you?

Jane: I don't know if I was accurate, I don't know what he means.

YA: So you, are you having…?

Jane: No, excuse me, I am not sure I understood what he said.

Josh: Oh, what I was saying is that, uh, at the moment that I said I was angry that's how I felt and then when, er, you…

Jane: Later on?

Josh: Yes, about a minute or so later, when you assessed that you didn't think I was, I think, er…

Jane: Oh, I get it…

Josh: I think that there had been enough change in the meantime that you were accurate.

Jane: I clued on to that part. Okay. I clued on to the last part that you weren't angry. That part.

Josh: Yeah, I had been…

Jane: So then…

Josh: A minute or two earlier but…

Jane: Yeah, okay…

YA: So how is that? You have had two different experiences, how is that for you? How is it for you to check out with another whether or not they have the experience that you *think* they are having? Is that hard for you?

Jane: I, I guess so. (*I let this 'guess' go by. I wish I hadn't!*)

YA: Okay. Is there anyone else in here who has that same difficulty? (*Al raises his hand.*) Yeah?

Al: Yes, when, because an awful lot of it is conflict, conflict between experience, with me…

YA: Yes?

Al: …experiences and moods are all in this direction (*gestures with his left hand*) thoughts that I have in my mind are all in that direction (*gestures with his right hand*).

Al's hand gestures clearly indicate the direction of his two 'forks': worries to the right, experience to the left. It is tempting to relate his 'experiences and moods' with his apprehensive right brain connection and his thoughts with his cognitive left brain.

YA: Yes.

Al: Which is in relationship to my physical tension. It can be very wearing.

YA: It pulls you in two different ways?

Al: Mmm.

YA: Yes, what is your experience right now, of sitting on the fence like you have been doing and hanging in there?

Al: Ah, just, just waiting to see if anything interests me, er, expectant, er, curious, er, interested, er, aroused emotionally slightly, but you pay for it. (*Negative prediction.*)

YA: Whoa! Whoa! You have just made a negative prediction, have you been paying for it so far?

Al: Well, yeah sure.

YA: Yes? How?

Al: With the conflicts between those emotions...

YA: Oh, I understand.

Al: ...and the thoughts.

YA: So you have been putting up with the pull.

Al: The payment, right.

YA: Has it been worth it?

Al: Uh.

YA: ...so far?

Al: I've always thought of it as being involuntary, so I never...I stopped asking myself whether it was worth it years ago...

Perhaps one of the major contributions that SCT makes to therapy is introducing the patient to the fact that there is a choice that can be made to withdraw their energy from their defensive anxiety-provoking thoughts and redirecting it towards exploring what experience they are defending against.

Al: ...because it was involuntary, uh, but I'd say no, it is not worth it ...(*indecipherable*) long time.

Keeping Al in the box

YA: So right this moment, I think you just went on to automatic there and answered the question the way you've answered it before rather than checking with your experience right here-and-now. Is that right?

Al: Yeah.

YA: Okay, so if you check with your experience about being in this group and sitting on the fence and paying attention and noticing that

> you felt curious and aroused, you noticed your experience then –
> and noticing that part of you had to compete with the part of
> you that is pulling you apart...

Al: I don't know...

YA: In this last half-hour has it been worth it or has it not?

Al: No, it hasn't been worth it.

YA: It hasn't been worth it.

Al: Not really.

YA: It hasn't been worth it?

Al: Not really.

YA: How do you feel about that, that somehow...

Al: I didn't...

YA: If you would...

Al: I have never had much experience...

YA: Take your time, take your time because if you answer too soon you're
not going to notice how you feel. Do you understand me?

The rhythm of personal time is an important issue in SCT. When a person is experiencing pressure to 'do it right' (working from their pre-programmed, adapted or defended self) they are tense, often anxious, their rhythm is faster, and their responses automatic – impulsive rather than spontaneous. Natural time, the inherent rhythm of curiosity and knowing, is different. Almost always it is slower, allowing information to come from exploring the experience of the moment. In short, information is accessed and processed differently by both the socialized self and the defensive self than when it is accessed and processed by the innate self. In SCT, the process of centering is designed to increase access to the experience of the innate self first (called the apprehensive self, in which experience is not primarily verbal) before the comprehensive self puts the experience into words.

In this part of the work, I am attempting to guide Al away from his defensive worrying towards his apprehensive experience. Feelings are not important in and of themselves in SCT. Rather the source that is generating the feelings is important.

> Al: It's all blocked up.

Choice

> YA: Wait! Whoa! If you answer too soon, you are not going to notice
> how you feel. Do you want to know how you feel? It's up to you
> (*pause*), it really is up to you right this moment.

Al: Yes.

YA: You want to?

Al: Yes.

YA: Okay, so how do you feel?

Al: Sad (*a poignant moment*).

Al buries his face in his right hand. I do not interrupt his moment of sad experience. From the SCT framework, pain at the cost of one's symptoms is the wedge that begins to transform symptoms from ego-syntonic to ego-dystonic. Thus, even though the therapist often also feels the pain for the person and for the human race (including his or her self), the pain is respected and framed empathically and harnessed to the work, rather than sympathized with.

YA: Yes. Sure. It really is sad how hard the work is to come into reality, isn't it? Is anyone else recognizing how hard the work is to come into reality and how strongly one wants to get pulled away?

(*Group members nod their heads with 'Yeah.'*)

YA: And sometimes one doesn't want to and sometimes one does. (*To June who is sitting relaxed and perhaps uninvolved.*) And you? Are you still sleepy?

June: No, I'm just so relaxed.

YA: Is that nice?

June: Very nice, I'm relaxed and listening to everybody.

YA: (*To Al*) Don't leave. Keep hanging on the fence there, okay, hanging on the fence. (*To June*) You've got the opportunity of learning more about what it's like to feel good.

June: Mmm.

Attempt to establish a 'feeling good' subgroup

This is an opportunity to increase June's access to her pleasure and to legitimize paying as much attention to the experience of pleasure in the group as to any of the other emotions. Getting the full experience of pleasure often gets short shrift in therapy. Indeed, not only in therapy – one can see the predisposition towards dissatisfaction and pain by the many words we have to describe it, and the relatively few we have for satisfaction and pleasure. However, June does not appear to be sufficiently focused to work.

YA: Is there anyone else feeling good? (*To Rose*) Yeah? You are? Good.

Rose: I've done a lot of that before too – the feeling one way and thinking the other way and I got sick and tired of paying for it and the struggle. It is tough to find, it was tough for me to find that my perception was not always reality.

YA: Just like...

Rose: That hurt...

YA: ...our friend here (*gesturing to Al*).

Rose: ...that hurt because it was really painful.

YA: Yes, so you were in the same boat there.

Jane: (*To Rose*) Mmm (*Rose looks towards Jane and nods*).

YA: And you're having, you're getting, both, an opportunity to open up to the experience of feeling good.

June: Mmm.

YA: (*To Al*) Which you can't feel just yet, can you? You can't feel good yet – hey! Come back!

Al: Yeah.

YA: You're sitting on the fence, remember? Don't let go because you know that you are sad and how strong the struggle is and you've also got two people here who, at the moment, aren't struggling and are having some pleasure.

Al: Mmm.

YA: Yes. You never can tell, it might work for you too.

Sam: (Joining Al's subgroup) It's possible. I just feel sad...

YA: Yes, sad about how hard it is?

Sam: I feel good that I am making the attempt, in fact.

Discrimination

YA: Right, so you're sad about how hard it is...

Sam: True.

YA: ...and glad that you are struggling.

Sam: Mmm (*nods*).

YA: (*To Al*) And you're just sad at how hard it is at the moment. (*To Al*) What is your name?

Al: Al.

YA: So at the moment (*to Al*), you are mostly sad at how hard it is?

Al: Yes (*nods*).

YA: (*To Sam*) And you're both sad at how hard it is now and glad that you are trying?

Sam: I'm hoping that in a year or two... (*indistinguishable*)

YA: You're probably right.

Sam: I hope so.

YA: The real world is rarely as hard as one thinks. (*To Rose*) And you are already feeling that you have got some mileage out of it? (*Rose nods*)

YA: And (*to June*) you are having a relatively new experience of being here?

Flight into person system

What follows is a very good example of what SCT calls 'flight into the person system.' This is a withdrawal of energy from the person's relationship to the context into the self-centered system, in which the self is the context. Thus, June does not join the work of the subgroup. The ideal is to have an awareness both of the self-centered system and the context outside the self which also generates experience.

June: I learned now how to be more positive instead of negative. I always thought negative, nothing ever was going to be right for me, nobody was ever going to like me, I don't know how to do anything right and now I'm learning. I look in the mirror and say to myself, 'You're beautiful, I love you.' I could never say that to myself. I felt silly the first time I did it but then I started feeling good about it 'cause I always downed myself and everything I did and then I would let everybody else around me down me and then I would go along and agree with them – 'You're right, you're right' – but here they're not right. I'm just as good as anybody else and I'm learning that now – to think of me first instead of worrying everybody around me.

YA: Is that what you did in this group?

June: Between being here and being in this group, listening to everybody but mainly listening to you.

YA: How was that?

June: It made me think I'm more important than anybody else – I'm number one and I'm going to stay number one. I'm not going to let them push me down to the ground no more.

YA: Well, if I might add, you're not going to let your thoughts push you down either.

June: Right and that's why I say I was so relaxed because I enjoyed
        everything you were saying and talking about and everything
        sunk in to what you were saying.

YA: So you had a good experience.

June: Uh-huh (*nodding her head*).

It seemed to me important not to work with June at this point, in that June's good
feelings are generated from a positive prediction about herself, and to bring her
into reality might have threatened her current accommodation. I had the
impression that she is significantly medicated and has been programmed into
positive thinking, which, provided she does not enter reality, will protect her from
her previous negative thinking. This is a different therapeutic approach from SCT
which requires members to increase their ability to accept both the good and bad
aspects of reality rather than splitting reactions into all good or all bad. A second
important reason is that time was running out.

Ending the group

YA: We have about ten minutes more and what I would suggest is that we
        talk a little bit about the experience that you have had in this
        group, what it's meant to you, what you're disappointed about
        and what maybe you're pleased about and whether you learned
        anything here. Would you take the next ten minutes just to say
        what your reactions are – whether you think this would be
        helpful, whether you think it wouldn't.

Driving and restraining forces

I am introducing a form of the exercise which is used in all SCT groups to facilitate
the transition from the work of the group to the reality outside the group – a
boundary that the members are about to cross. The exercise calls for 'surprises–
learnings–satisfactions–dissatisfactions and discoveries.' Satisfactions and dissatisfactions are particularly important as they can be made operational for the next
steps in work. Satisfactions are the driving forces that connect the members to
their goal, and dissatisfactions are the restraining forces that get in the way of
reaching that goal. Members are therefore encouraged to do more of what satisfies
them, and to do one thing less that led to their dissatisfaction.

I am actually introducing the spirit of the force field even if I am not explicitly
introducing the technique (see Chapter 3, p.100).

Bill: I'm a little disappointed 'cause I can't feel any emotion around.

YA: Yes.

Bill: I don't feel anything.

YA: Yes. So history repeated itself with you.

Bill: Yes. And if I went back up to my room, I probably could lay down and cry for a half hour. I'm disappointed I can't – like I said before, I see my therapist every week.

I am encouraging Bill to bring his disappointment into the context of reality. In reality he can set a goal (crying) and can get a sense of whether he is approaching it or avoiding it.

Weakening the restraining forces

YA: Let me try again. See the useful thing about disappointment – the useful thing about disappointment is to see what you could do so that you don't get so disappointed again. So when is your next therapy session?

Bill: Outpatient? Inpatient? In a half hour – in a half hour.

YA: So would you like to bring your feelings into your group in a half hour?

Bill: (*Inaudible.*)

YA: No, no that's not what I asked you.

Bill: Would I like to? Yes.

YA: Okay, so can you think of one thing that you did in here this afternoon that made it harder for you to bring your feelings in, which is what you want to do – one thing that you would be able to change in a half hour. (*Bill shrugs.*) If you shrug you're not going to be really engaged in the conflict and find out what is the one thing, one thing that you did in here this afternoon which if you *don't do* it in a half hour you have a better chance of bringing your feelings in, which is what you want to do.

I am continuing to introduce the force field into the group.

Bill: Probably it's to try...to try to interact in the group, in the next group we're going to, in the same way I do when I'm all by myself.

YA: Okay, and how would that be different? What would you do differently if you interacted in the group the same way that you do when you're by yourself?

Bill: (*Long pause, sighs*) I don't know, I...for years... (*He is about to launch into his story-telling defense.*)

YA: Not for years. (*I re-orient him back to 'now'.*) In half-an-hour we start to...

Bill: I don't...

Establishing the goal for change

YA: Yes you do, so let's hang in there – what would be one thing you could do differently in the group in a half hour so that you have a better chance of doing what you want to do, which is to bring your feelings in?

Bill: Yes. Just be honest.

YA: And so what would you do honestly in a half hour in the group that you didn't do in here?

Bill: I'd talk about my feelings, I would feel...

YA: As you are talking?

Bill: As I'm talking.

YA: Yes, okay.

Bill: I don't feel – I talk *about* my feelings.

Insight

I would not have predicted that Bill would be one of the members to get an important insight. If Bill can keep that insight, he will have identified his major defense that prevents him from working in therapy – 'talking about' his feelings rather than learning about his experience of them.

YA: Right, okay, I understand. So in a half hour would you do your best to connect having your feelings first and your words second. See if that works. (*Bill nods and says 'mmm.'*) That would be the other way around.

Bill: Yes.

YA: Anybody else surprised or disappointed or...?

Rose: I found this to be a very...

YA: (*Interrupts*) He's falling off the fence – don't let him fall off the fence. (*Sam shakes Al's leg to bring him back.*)

YA: I'm sorry – go ahead.

Rose: I found this to be very interesting because I think that I've been doing a lot of reading about the sort of thing that you did in here but I have not really seen anybody do what you did before. I've been in many different group sessions because...

YA: If you explain you won't explore your experience right now.

The word 'because' almost always leads to an explanation of experience that diverts attention from exploring the experience.

> Rose: Uh-huh. You showed me how to focus more on what's happening at this point in time. Plus your way of doing so was quite different than any other therapist I've seen before because you were a bit stronger which I feel is necessary, but you did that with compassion. And attempting to take a group of people, many who don't know one another, and within one hour accomplishing a sense of community, is almost an impossible task – but I saw a point in there where you went over that hurdle and I felt it was a very useful group for me to be in – and I thank you for it.

Strengthening the driving forces

> YA: Do you know one thing that you did today that took you in the direction that you want to go, that you would want to do more of?
>
> Rose: Even more focusing on...focusing on right now.
>
> YA: Okay. (*We smile at each other.*) Anyone else?
>
> Sam: I have a problem.
>
> YA: What's that?
>
> Sam: What I learned from you is that you kind of force people – without all the gingerbread – to concentrate on this five minutes or this ten minutes, don't go off...
>
> YA: That's true.
>
> Sam: A lot of the other groups I've gone to, you know, they let you ramble on and on about what your problems are in the future and what got you here and what we're doing right now is what will eventually get us out of here. And you hung right in there.

Unfinished business

> YA: And the unfinished business that you and I had was that we didn't finish confronting whether you were going to go your way or whether you were going to try to go my way. And it seems to me that that's a very important place for you to be, solidly helping yourself and not pleasing me.

Sam: Pleasing you is not going to help me.

YA: Right – that's right, pleasing you is going to help you.

Sam: That's the main thing, to hell with the next hour and a half (*makes a gesture indicating here-and-now*).

YA: Right, 'cause the moment that we're living is right now, isn't it?

Rose: (*Joking with YA*) I told him that last night, but he didn't listen to me.

YA: (*Joking back*) Well I'm in the chair where people listen more easily!

Sam: You hold... You're in this group like I said, you didn't let her off the hook (*looking at Jane*). You made her confront her feelings.

YA: And you liked that?

Sam: Yes.

Rose: Strong stuff, good stuff!

YA: Anybody else got any disappointments or surprises or satisfactions or learnings?

Nan: I'm disappointed in myself.

YA: Well, let's see if we can turn that disappointment into your next step. What would you like to have done here that you didn't?

Nan: Open up and be able to spill my feelings.

From an SCT point of view 'spilling feelings' for Nan is probably the least therapeutic thing for her to do. Learning to recognize the difference between the feelings that are generated either from thoughts or regression, and the feelings that are connected to experience in the realities of herself and her environment, would be the major focus of SCT therapy. However, in this part of the group, I am introducing members to the idea that they have some choice about what they can do more of and what they can do less of. Therefore I accept whatever their satisfaction of dissatisfaction is.

Putting Nan in the box

YA: Okay, and can you notice one thing that you did that made that more difficult for you?

Nan: I put my wall up (*again, a phrase that has the flavor of 'being programmed in a previous therapy*).

YA: Okay, and how do you do that?

Nan: Just shut everybody out.

YA: No, no, no. Excuse me, but *how* do you do that, how do you build your wall?

Nan: By not letting nobody in.

YA: Well, how do you do that?

Nan: Eh...

YA: Do you think things, do you feel things?

Nan: I think things, I think...

YA: What?

Nan: Like I'm not going to get close, I'm not going to get involved.

YA: So, you program yourself?

Nan: Uh-huh.

YA: Okay, and when is your next therapy session?

Nan: I'm not sure.

YA: Aren't you?

Nan: No, I just got here Saturday.

YA: What?

Nan: I just got here Saturday.

YA: So you're not in a group?

Nan: No.

YA: Not yet?

Nan: Not yet.

YA: Okay, you're going to be in a group some time this week?

Nan: I should be.

YA: Okay, so when you go into that group, one of the things that you might try is every time you start to program yourself, you tell the group, I'm programming myself and putting the wall up and I don't want to do that.

Nan: Okay.

YA: Would you try that?

Nan: Yes I will, thank you, thank you.

YA: Because of course it's disappointing if you do the same thing over and over but it's less disappointing if you know what you're doing, because then, even though it's very painful as we know from you (*looking at Al*) ...are you on the fence? Or have you dropped out?

Al: Mostly, on.

YA: Okay. What we're working with right now is exactly what you are working with – which is change, it is so difficult, it is so hard to struggle against the old habits and if you don't struggle against the old habits then you do the same thing over again (*long pause in the group*). Anyone else, satisfied – yes?

Josh: No, I'm disappointed.

YA: Yes?

Josh: Also with myself.

YA: What is it *you* would like to have done differently?

Josh: Well, I've got a glimpse of the state that you're trying to get us to reach and a couple of the people have said they did reach it and I'm not sure what your purpose is but I see a value in it and it's as you said, but I'm not able so far to get anywhere, and it feels good.

YA: So, did you notice any things that you did today that may have slowed you up?

Josh: It's hard to say because I'm trying so to go to a certain place and I can't see what direction it is, and I'm searching in all directions for explanations, methods, whatever, but I don't see anything useful.

From the SCT perspective, Josh has exactly the opposite therapeutic challenge from Nan. Whereas with Nan it would be important to help her make the boundary less permeable between her feelings and her thoughts, with Josh it would be important to make the boundary more permeable, in that he filters all experience through his cognitive intelligence at the expense of his emotional intelligence.

YA: Okay, so what I would say is that there's always a fork in the road between explaining things and exploring things.

Josh: I couldn't see it, don't see that.

YA: Yes, I understand that. But maybe when you have the opportunity, when it feels right for you, if you would hold the explanations aside for awhile and just see what you discover instead, at some time when it feels right for you, you try that. Explore your experience instead of explaining it. And maybe you can get help to learn how to do that?

Josh: Yeah.

YA: Anybody else? We're sort of coming to the end of our time right now (*pause*). Okay, well, thank you very, very, very much, for what you have done with me today, and I really do thank you. We have just had our first experience of using this method in hospital. And if we did it again, would you want to come back?

(*Members all nod and say 'yes.'*)

Rose: Very, very much so.

YA: Would you? Well, thank you very, very much indeed.

Rose: Thank you.

Nan: I enjoyed it, I really did.

Rose: We don't want to leave! (*joking with YA*)

Pam: I'm sorry I was late. The doctor had precedent...

YA: That was something you didn't have a choice about.

Pam: No, I didn't. But from what I've picked up, I've worked in groups like this before, but I have to say you were the sternest, er, mediator, or facilitator.

YA: Did you have a feeling about that?

Pam: Oh yes.

YA: What was it?

Pam: Eh, the other groups I've been in, if you were the facilitator, you wouldn't have gone on for 18 or 20 weeks, we would have been done in two or three because, like you say, you have explanations go on too long, it's the exploring that does the good – and the group would have struggled on for ever and ever with all the explanations, so had you been my facilitator I wouldn't have spent so much money in counseling, thank you.

YA: Thank you.

It is important, in SCT, to cross the boundary out of an ending group with a clear 'goodbye.' This gives the opportunity for members verbally to recognize the separation, and also to be reminded that it is only the present goodbye that is generating their feelings, and not to import their past, more difficult goodbyes. As you will see, however, I didn't do it. Thus, both at the beginning and ending of this group, I failed to set the SCT boundaries. I can only say that at the beginning of the group I was nervous, and at this ending I was very sad that I would not be working with this particular group and these particular members again. There is often a cost in not following the SCT guidelines. Mine was that the group and its members are still with me.

The members said goodbye and thank you as they left the room. It was reported to me later that they remained talking outside on the grass for another 20 minutes before they separated and went back to their wards.

Feedback

The final important question was whether the positive feelings that the members ended the group with would carry over time. We collected feedback from the members two days later. The feedback from eight of the nine members was as follows:

- I viewed this as a therapist creating a breath of fresh air. I felt that the experience was opening me up. It was refreshing.

- This group was more direct. The focus was on what we were trying to accomplish. It was a now meeting – what is happening now.

- Her types of meeting wouldn't have wasted as much time as lots of other groups I have been in.

- I thought it was wonderful. Got lots of positives about myself. Took a look at myself. Way she went about trying to open people made me feel good. I got insight on things like why I am here.

- ...knowledge that living in present is best way to live. If you spend all time in the past you miss the present.

- It was condensed, not (*indecipherable*) focused. I didn't tell my life story (*indecipherable*). I got nothing personally, but have been in a group before. Trying to learn lesson about staying in present.

- If all therapists could work this way it would save time. The therapist was tough, she interrupted me three times.

- What she was trying to do was hard for me to actually do. I can think it is plausible to do if done with high frequency, three times a week would be useful. With outpatients once a week it would be dramatically harder. It took me the whole hour to get the directions she was trying to point me to. Just the whole idea of focusing on current feeling rather than thinking about them or the past or the future. If you can do that several times in row would be useful. I don't have an opinion about whether it is valuable. It was hard to do for me.

Notes

1   Theoretically, information is energy which is available for work, and ambiguity, contradiction or redundancy in communications act like noise and make it less likely that the information in the communication will get through. Whenever leaders have information that the group has not, they have more autonomy than the group has. This is by no means unusual in a group and is typically reinforced by the power and control that the group usually gives to the leader in a group. The question is, does the leader keep the power and control to him or herself or transfer it to the group? Another SCT goal is to transfer information about how to manage oneself in one's environment as soon as the group is able to use it. You will see examples of this as I first establish the

comfort of functional subgrouping and then proceed to 'educate' the group that anxiety does not come 'out of the blue' but has three recognizable sources and can be modified.

2 SCT considers story-telling a particularly pernicious defense in group therapy. The cost on the members is that it allows them to stay in the oft-told tale which fixates them in the familiar past (even when told with great emotion) and prevents them from discovering how the present is different from the past. The cost on the group-as-a-whole is that it establishes a 'flight' norm.

I make a bid to re-orient the group towards functional subgrouping by turning towards the members who are supporting my lead. This is one of the SCT paradoxes: the SCT goal is to enable members to become researchers of their own experience so that they can choose to 'discover' themselves. Yet, by setting the structure, the SCT leader 'boxes members in' so that they have no choice but to explore their experience rather than explain it.

3 Generalizing interventions are designed to legitimize, humanize, normalize and depathologize human experience.

4 Habib Davanloo (1987), in his training tapes, demonstrates the difference between when there is 'life' in the hands of the person talking and when there is not. He cautions that pressure should not be put on the defenses of those whose hands and body are not engaged. Not only are they not 'present' to engage in work, but they may also be disconnected in a more serious way. In contrast, Dr. Davanloo claims that pressure on the defenses can be safely applied when there is 'life' (central nervous system involvement) in the person's hands.

5 It is interesting to note that Jane's individual therapist counted her as one of his most difficult group patients outside the hospital.

6 Connecting parallel talk to the underlying group theme becomes important when the group is becoming aware of the group-as-a-whole as a third context for understanding their work. The SCT expectation is that the group theme will surface when the defenses in the group-as-a-whole are sufficiently modified. The same is true of assocations.

7 I felt surprise and relief when the group did validate my summary in that it gave me some confidence that I was validating the process of teaching how to validate reality rather than induce compliance.

8 Technically, in a more experienced group, this would be an opening to use the format of the distraction exercise which requires members to give the facts of their distraction first, and their feelings second, thus giving both the member and the leader an opportunity to ascertain whether the feelings are coming from fact or from thoughts. Managing hallucinations in an SCT group is not different from managing any other distraction that keeps the member's energy out of the group. It appears to be surprisingly reassuring to members to work with their hallucinations in the same format as other members do their distractions and dreams.

9 The observing self-system in SCT is different from the observing ego, in that it is developed to enable the discrimination of differences, and thus pave the way for the ongoing work of first exploring differences and then integrating them, which leads to being able to understand differing levels of complexity in experiences.

10 It is tempting to connect the split between Al's defensive thoughts and his reality experience with his hand gestures and their assumed connection to the right brain and left brain. He uses his right hand to indicate when he 'checks out' reality – collects

data, sees what's going on – all cognitive left brain functions(?). His checking out is generated by curiosity (a right brain function(?)). With access to both the emotional stimulus of curiosity and the cognitive ability to collect data, he has all the raw material for functioning with emotional intelligence with which he would then be able to solve his problems. However, he uses his left hand (right brain) to indicate his obsessive worries (which he can 'put down' briefly when he is curious). It can be argued that he blocks his right brain knowledge by his defensive worrying. The SCT 'fork in the road' technique is the method that enables people to restore their ability to discriminate and integrate cognitive and emotional knowledge. This is demonstrated when Al, much later in the script, says he feels sad for himself.

11   Here again, a member's experience is related to both himself and the work of the group, identifying the common theme from earlier group work to help create common bonds among the members.

12   It is important to note, however, that to open the process to questions and answers in response to a defiant or compliant question reinforces non-functional dependence.

13   While Josh and I are in interaction, the microphone cord, which has slipped off my shoulder, is being adjusted by a technician. I am astonished, watching the tape, that neither I nor the group are distracted by this. This is a good criterion on which to assess how focused on work a group is. I remember teaching a class in group dynamics once when fireman, in full regalia, entered the room, checking to see if there was a fire, and the group continued working on its task without breaking attention!

14   Here is another good example of how group members, by their discovery of their own defenses, reinforce the SCT techniques (which were largely developed by tracing the spontaneous emergence of the sequence of defenses that occur in development phases of a group).

15   Systems survive, develop from simple to complex, and transform through the process of discriminating differences and integrating them.

16   Functional dependency is dependency which allows the group to co-operate with the leader in the direction of the group goals, compliantly and at the same time involved authentically.

CHAPTER THREE

The Techniques of Systems-Centered Therapy

All group therapies have methods for resolving the conflicts and directing the work energy of the group. What is different in the systems-centered approach is that the methods and techniques for both activities are introduced from the very first few moments of a group, in a step by step hierarchy from the simplest and easiest to the more complex and difficult.

There are two kinds of human responses generic to all groups that are modified immediately in a systems-centered group. First is the inherent human tendency to split away from unacceptable differences (in the self as well as in others). In SCT, this is contained by introducing functional subgrouping. The second is the defensive use of language that is designed to manage closeness and distance between people, rather than to exchange information that is related to the work that people have come together to do. In SCT, addressing the kinds of defensive communications that members bring into the group is done by 'boundarying.'

Initiation into systems-centered methods in all new groups begins immediately with an introduction of subgrouping around a common experience (for the inpatient group in Chapter 2, the common experience was working in a fishbowl (a circle in the middle with observers around – and for our group, the addition of lights and cameras!)). Subgrouping around a common experience initiates a supportive climate in which members come to rely on not being left out on a limb to work alone.

Technically, functional subgrouping is an essential first step in establishing a method for discriminating and integrating differences instead of denying or attacking them.[1] It is this human aversion to differences which manifests itself in the overt and covert scapegoating in groups that led me to postulate that 'the only dynamic that was important to the survival and development of living human systems was the ability to recognize and integrate differences' (Agazarian 1997). As the techniques of functional subgrouping developed, it became apparent that in fact, although the underlying human impulse to scapegoat differences remained the same, exploring the impulse instead of acting on it made a very big difference to the way members worked together and to the developmental potential of the group-as-a-whole.

As soon as subgrouping is established, SCT immediately addresses the distancing language that is used to maintain separate and stereotypical relationships rather than to join and establish working relationships. The obvious example of distancing communication is the concealed disagreement in the 'yes, but,' in which the 'yes' is a token joining and the 'but' a separation. A 'yes, but' pattern of communication is a socially acceptable way to argue. A less obvious form of social control is the use of questions. Leading questions and narrow questions control the direction of the communication; personal questions control personal communication; fact-finding questions control the kind of information that is introduced. 'Why' questions direct the communication into explanations. On the other hand, 'what,' 'where,' 'how' and 'when' questions reduce the ambiguity, contradictions and redundancy in the communication.

The kind of defensive communication that makes it difficult to understand or be understood is like background noise which drowns out the information in the message (Shannon and Weaver 1964). It makes common sense that 'noisy' communication serves as a restraining force to 'clear' communication, and that simply reducing noise simultaneously increases clarity and understanding.[2]

In SCT groups, the tendency that human beings have to control themselves and others through the way they use language is modified immediately by both subgrouping and boundarying. The methods of functional subgrouping and boundarying will be addressed in more detail in this chapter after some of the less formalized techniques have been discussed.

There is a lot for systems-centered members to learn informally in the beginning of a systems-centered group. They have to learn the 'language' – not just the new words, but new ways of understanding basic facts about their world that had been previously taken for granted. As you may have noticed in the script, the more formal introduction of the methods of subgrouping and boundarying that form the major theme from the beginning of the group is interspersed with 'asides' that introduce techniques like the force field, the 'fork in the road of choice,' 'the edge of the unknown,' 'turbulence at the boundary,' 'reframing' and understanding 'time travel' so that members can discriminate between the past, the present and the future. These 'asides' make it possible to work at two levels at once.

Past + Present + the future

Fork in the road

The 'fork in the road of choice' is a basic SCT technique (Agazarian 1997). It is the technique that connects the group and its members to their goals. Its advantage is that it is an immediate orientation to many of the SCT values. First and foremost it presents the paradox of choice. On the one hand, the patient is free to choose whichever side of the conflict he or she wants to explore first. On the other hand, the patient has no choice about whether or not to choose.

For example, the first choice introduced into a new group is the choice between exploring an experience and explaining it. By exploring the impulse to explain, members discover that explaining leads them to what they know already. Exploring experience leads them to what they don't know. Discovering the unknown is, of course, the goal of therapy. If you explain, you will lead yourself to what you know already. There is an alternative fork in the road, and that is to explore the experience that you are having right now that you are attempting to explain! Test it out, and see whether it is true that 'explaining' takes you to your thoughts whereas exploring leads you to your experience.

As the fork in the road requires patients to 'observe' their defensive constella-tions in order to explore their significance and cost, and to explore their own unknown to discover what conflict, sensation, emotion or impulse they are defending against, it is extremely important that fork in the road intervention is made in a way that arouses curiosity rather than resistance. The more an intervention makes common sense, the more likely it is that it will arouse co-operation rather than defiance or compliance.

The fork in the road technique gives members a choice as to which side of the conflict they wish to explore first. The following is taken from my work with Al's ambivalence (all ambivalence is reframed as a defense against conflict which disappears when the conflict is identified).

> Al says: 'Sitting on the fence and not wanting to make a commitment to putting my chips down in any particular spot...' I reply: 'Yeah, but you know, sitting on the fence is a very good place to be, to look down the forks in the road. When you are sitting on the fence like that, you begin to have a choice about whether you want to take yourself further out of the group or whether you want to bring yourself further into the group.' (see p.67)

Using the fork in the road technique, members are consistently required to search for and experience the active conflict that underlies passive defensive cognitions like ambivalence or cognitive distortions. Discriminating and integrating infor-mation is a never-ending process, and using the fork in the road application, manages the tendency in all groups to regress when chaotic or unconcious material threatens to emerge in the group by progressively exploring, discov-ering, discriminating and integrating unfamiliar information as it arises in the group.

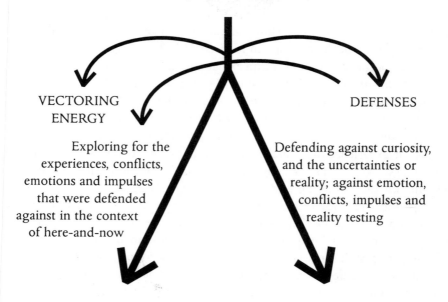

Defense Modification
THE FORK IN THE ROAD
Between exploring experience and defending
against experience

VECTORING
ENERGY

DEFENSES

Exploring for the
experiences, conflicts,
emotions and impulses
that were defended
against in the context
of here-and-now

Defending against curiosity,
and the uncertainties or
reality; against emotion,
conflicts, impulses and
reality testing

Figure 3.1 The fork in the road

Figure 3.1, the picture of the fork in the road, illustrates how the energy that is bound up in defenses is released when the defense is undone. The energy is then available for exploring what conflict, impulse or emotion is being defended against. The fork in the road uses the same principle of change as the force field that is discussed below.

The force field

The force field is a model developed by Kurt Lewin (1951) that can be understood simply through common sense. If one reduces the restraining forces that lie along the path to the system's goal, the system's driving forces will automatically be released to move in the direction of the goal. The balance of driving and restraining forces determines how much energy or information is available for work. All the methods of systems-centered practice are designed to release the drive by reducing the restraining forces that inhibit it.

The force field equivalent of the fork in the road is represented in Table 3.1.

Table 3.1 Force field of driving and restraining forces in relationship to defensive and non-defensive experience

Force field model	
Exploring experience ⟶	⟵ Defending against experience
Exploring before explaining ⟶	⟵ Explaining before exploring
Accepting uncertainty ⟶	⟵ Being certain
Testing reality ⟶	⟵ Taking reality for granted
Being curious ⟶	⟵ Being incurious

Adapting the force field into the work of therapy has had a significant impact on the management of change. It is clear that weakening the restraining forces is a great deal more efficient than attempting to increase the driving forces. There is a simple way to experience this. Make fists and position them so that they push against each other. You will find that however much you increase the force in your right fist you do not manage to move your left fist, and however hard you push with your left fist you do not move your right. This is an example of equal and opposite forces maintaining the equilibrium of the moment. Attempting to push against resistance requires a greater force than is usually available. Now, as you keep up the pressure, suddenly weaken one wrist. You will find that your other fist drives forward with free force. You have now experienced the systems-centered method, which is to intervene to weaken the restraining forces and free the drive within all living human systems so that it can be directed towards the working goal. As will be discussed later, SCT systematically weakens defenses in a predefined hierarchy. These defenses serve as restraining forces to the development of the group. Thus, by systematically reducing the defenses, the individual members gain access to their innate drive towards survival and development and the group is enabled through the phases of its development.

Reframing

In the practice of SCT, how feelings are generated is taken very seriously. Feeling language can be simple or complex. Simple feeling words are a direct translation of emotion, using words like fear, anger, grief and joy. Complex feeling words combine a feeling experience with a thought about it and can serve either to code experience or to frame it. 'Feeling guilty,' for example, codes a conflict in experience between the emotion that is experienced and the opinion that it should not be. Complex feeling words like 'abandoned' or 'rejected' interpret experience. Words like abandoned, rejected and indealized are good examples of 'frames' in that they frame, classify or interpret a complex experience. Once the interpretation is framed in a word *it generates experience.*

There is no question that finding the right word to frame an experience serves an important function in that it both contains and communicates the emotional meaning of the original experience. It is very satisfying when the words match the music, even if the music is sad. However, problems arise immediately when a 'look-alike' complex event is immediately framed in terms of a past interpretation; it is the frame that generates the feelings and not the current experience. Framing is yet another automatic behavior that we humans use to explain or interpret an event rather than explore the reality of our experience. In SCT, it is immediately brought to the members' attention *when* they have framed (interpreted) their experience, and that their feelings are coming from their interpretation, not the underlying experience. They are then asked to discover the emotional response that they defended against by framing it. It is important to note that by adopting a frame, like 'abandoned' or 'rejected,' the member has automatically taken on the victim role.

A major technique, and one of the most powerful in SCT practice, is reframing. SCT therapists take every opportunity to normalize, depathologize, humanize and universalize the dynamics that are so often given bad press in the group (Agazarian 1997). Thus anxiety at not knowing what is going to happen next is reframed as normal apprehension at the edge of the unknown. Shyness or embarrassment in revealing oneself is reframed as turbulence at the boundary. This reframe is designed to establish a norm of accepting the experience as a normal part of human experience – a fork in the road between paying attention to the turbulence or to what one is wanting to communicate.

> Whenever we bring ourselves in, it is always a little embarrassing, we are always a little bit shy, sometimes we are a little bit ashamed, sometimes we are a lot. But if we pay attention to the embarrassment and the shame and the shyness, we won't be able to bring ourselves in, and if we pay attention more to the wish to bring ourselves in, we have got a better chance. So you are at another fork in the road: if you pay attention to your shame, it is going to be harder for you to bring yourself in *now* (see p.71).

Discriminations in reframing

One of the most important aspects of reframing is continually bringing discriminations to members' awareness. For example, feelings that are generated by thoughts may feel the same, but they are not the same as feelings generated by emotional experience.

In SCT, feelings are defined as different from emotion. Emotion is essentially a nonverbal experience. Emotions are communicated nonverbally (the spontaneous

[margin handwritten note, left side:] Framing or interpreting my experience – it is the frame that generates the feelings + not the current experience

[margin handwritten note, top right:] RE-FRAMING

smile or frown) or through intention movements (the clenched fist, the shrug). Emotions must be translated into feelings before they can be communicated verbally. In SCT, therefore, emotion is discriminated from feeling in that emotion is an experience without words, and feeling is the experience after emotion has been translated into words. SCT lays great emphasis on subgrouping to explore rather than defend against or act out emotional 'intentions,' making the assumption that translating emotion into words contains it.

When feelings serve as a direct translation of emotion then the person is engaged in the process of discriminating and integrating their experience: sometimes discovering new emotional depths, sometimes gaining emotional insight, sometimes finding words to fit their experience.[3]

For example, a very important SCT discrimination is made around guilt which leads to both a different understanding and a different response to the experience once the common sense discriminations have been made. SCT frames guilt as a collision between the thought about what 'ought to be' and the fact of 'what is.' Accepting the reality that what is, *is*, and separating the reality from the thought that it *should be* different, makes room for the recognition of the feelings underlying guilt, which are sometimes remorse and regret, and at other times are discovered to be triumph or pleasure or satisfaction (whether they 'ought to be' or not). This is a good example of how the frame (in this case, the word 'guilt') can serve as a substitute for the real experience and generate feelings that may or may not be connected to the current experience.

Another important reframe arises from discriminating the components of a universal human emotion, like yearning. Members most often experience yearning as painful. This pain arises from a failure to separate out the experience of wanting from the remembered experience of not getting. The pain comes from memories of disappointments, not from the experience of wanting. When the discrimination is made, the actual experience of wanting is nearly always discovered to be a deep, fulfilling and motivating experience.

The consequence of making the kinds of discriminations that lead to a reframing of experience is that it enables a shift from a passive victim experience to a proactive state. To use the example of 'abandonment' again, the frame is often, unfortunately, accepted or even interpreted in therapy in such a way that it becomes a substitute for reality. When members are encouraged to explore underneath the frame, they discover a complex range of feelings: perhaps anger at not having the relationship or situation that they wished, perhaps pain at the disappointment, perhaps fear at the uncertainty of the alternatives and, often, some courage, resourcefulness and determination to help themselves. They discover that each 'look-alike' event of being 'abandoned' has a different emotional mix, and a different emotional impact when it is explored instead of simply framed.

Another important discrimination made in SCT is to separate out the experience of an emotion from its target. The example below is about rage, but it is equally true for other emotions, like love or hate or grief. The connection to the 'target' is personal, the basic emotion is existential.

> Sam: I've got some anger at myself.
>
> YA: Let's separate out the experience of the feeling of anger and how you target it.
>
> Sam: Okay.
>
> YA: Because one can have anger and one can target it in all sorts of different ways. One can target it at oneself, one can target it at me, one can target it at the world. But what about the feeling of anger? Have you got a feeling of anger? (see pp.75–76)

Later, when angry impulses to retaliate against others in sadistic ways emerge, they are depathologized as a universal human response to being frustrated or thwarted. Of course, acknowledging the universality of normal human dynamics increases the likelihood that the fantasies, fears and impulses that can horrify and terrify members will be explored in subgroups rather than labeled as sick, dangerous or bad. Another advantage is that it makes it easier for members to recognize that they tend to project onto and into others the aspects of themselves that they are pathologizing.[4]

Discrimination and integration are basic to the theory of living human systems, the source of the method of functional subgrouping. SCT assumes that it is through the development of the ability to discriminate and integrate that systems survive, develop and transform. Whenever there is an opportunity, therefore, the process is reinforced by drawing the member's (and the group's) attention to the discriminations that they are making without knowing it, doing no more than preparing the ground for later work.

Sam says, 'I am a little nervous about being here, but I figure, anything that can help…it's worth giving it a try.' I point out that he has 'two realities and one wish.'

Discriminations are also, of course, fundamental to identifying subgroups: 'We have a subgroup here where the unknown is not knowing what is going to happen here… And in a sense, for you, your unknown is you don't know what is happening inside you.' (see pp.47–48)

Perhaps the most important discrimination made in systems-centered therapy is the fact that feelings are generated from different sources, and it is important to recognize which source is generating them, particularly as people tend to 'act on their feelings' whether they are grounded in fantasy or in the reality of emotional experience.

In SCT, it is immediately brought to the members' attention when they have used a frame to describe their experience, and they are asked to check and see if it is the frame that is now generating their experience. If it is, they are then asked to discover what their emotional response was to the event that they defended against by framing it and by taking refuge in the victim role.

Time travel

All groups begin with behavior that is characteristic of intellectual flight – flight from the here-and-now of the present into the past or the future (see Table 3.3, p.119). Diagnosing flight from the present is simply a matter of listening for a change of tense. 'I am' signals experience in the present, 'I will' signals a journey into the future, and 'I was' a journey into the past. In SCT we call this time traveling.

It is often a new idea that one can deliberately direct and focus one's energy 'across boundaries' into the here-and-now. SCT members learn that there are psychological boundaries that structure the space and time of mental reality, just as there are real boundaries in space and time. Coming to recognize mental time and space boundaries make it possible for members to notice how they 'go' and where they go. That this is new and difficult learning is clear from how hard the patients worked to grasp the concept of the here-and-now, and how much harder they had to work to put it into practice. This is well illustrated in one of the member's feedback collected two days after the group experience:

> What she was trying to do was hard for me to actually do. I can think it is plausible to do if done with high frequency, three times a week would be useful. With outpatients once a week it would be dramatically harder. It took me the whole hour to get the directions she was trying to point me to. Just the whole idea of focusing on current feeling rather than thinking about them or the past or the future. If I can do that several times in a row would be useful. Don't have opinion about whether it is valuable. It was hard for me to do. (see p.94)

In our experience in SCT we take it for granted that everybody 'time travels.' As one of our patients said: 'When you leave the here-and-now you can go anywhere!' One of the first discoveries for SCT members is that they can learn to tell when going to the past or the future is flight from the work in the present and when it is useful to their present work. We have learned to take it for granted that for almost all new members in SCT training groups it comes as a surprise to discover that they can *choose* which time dimension they wish to live in. It is no surprise then, that the patients in this group were no wiser than the general population.

There are several very good examples from the inpatient group of how foreign it is to people to deliberately come into the present.

> Bill: Fine. I just wiped out the fact there's – I know there's a camera here and I know there's people over there, but I'm oblivious to it.

YA: So how are you, being in the group with us? Do you have a feeling about that?

Bill: A feeling about that? I am just wondering how I am going to react when we start interacting with each other.

Rose: I am just here.

YA: Okay. No feeling yet?

Rose: There's nothing to have a feeling of. Because I don't know what is going to happen, so how can I make a judgment about it? I am just waiting to see. (see pp.49–50)

Characteristic of all these responses is the idea that the present must stimulate a reaction *before* it exists. The SCT alternative is to learn to tell the difference between one's experience from past or future associations, and being open to one's internal experience in the context of ones 'here-and-now' self in the present.

The major restraining force to being aware of the present is that it is, in reality, uncertain. Living in the present means living at the edge of the unknown, which is why it is one of the first issues to be addressed in SCT, and why people are encouraged to be curious so that their energy goes towards exploring rather than explaining prematurely.

The edge of the unknown

Being at the 'edge of the unknown' is another important concept in SCT. It is the apprehensive experience of being in uncertainty, often contaminated with dread and anxiety about not knowing what is going to happen next. When curiosity about the unknown is mobilized, anxiety is often transformed into excitement, anticipation and wonder, which is the state labeled 'apprehension at the edge of the unknown.' You will see that I take the first opportunity to reinforce this when I say to June: 'So you are right at the edge of the unknown in a sense.' June responds with: 'It's new and I'm curious!' This gives me the opportunity to reinforce her contribution to the group: 'Well, what I find is if I go into something new and I am a little anxious, being curious is really helpful.'

I also take the opportunity to legitimize uncertainty as a useful experience when I say to Sam: 'So you are also on the edge of the unknown...and curious?' And later to Jane: 'And is it also for you that it is right on the edge of the unknown?' And then to Josh (with a discrimination): 'And in a sense, your unknown is you don't know what is happening inside you.'

Formal SCT methods: Subgrouping and boundarying

In contrast to, perhaps, all other approaches to group psychotherapy, the formal methods that make an SCT group are introduced as soon as the group begins.

Unlike an indirect approach, in which the group norms emerge gradually from the way that its members interact with each other, and unlike the direct approach where members' behavior is modified *after* it is brought into the group, SCT modifies behavior immediately, *before* it becomes established as a norm in the group, by shaping communication as soon as it crosses the boundary into the group (boundarying) and at the same time establishing functional subgrouping, so that no member has to work alone while group behavior is being shaped (Agazarian 1997).

Thus it is that every new group starts by learning how to work in a subgroup. Subgrouping provides the method for containing the conflicts and problems that lie on the path to goal so that they can be addressed in a way that reduces rather than increases them. Boundarying provides the methods for managing noise (defensive communications) that would disrupt the system. Boundarying accomplishes this task by reducing the restraining forces of ambiguity, contradiction and redundancy.

As always, structure (boundarying) and function (subgrouping) are interdependent. The group's first steps into functional subgrouping manage conflicts over differences and at the same time direct communication across the boundaries in a self-correcting (boundarying) and goal-directed (vectoring) way. For example, as members learn the difference between 'waving, pushing and rowing' communications (see p.108), they also learn that 'rowing' requires giving up explaining, questioning or interpreting others so that they can explore their experience instead.[5] Explaining and interpreting are on the road to what is known already, exploring is the road to the unknown. Thus in the context of subgrouping, not only is discrimination and integration of information modified but so is the organization of information (energy) in self-correcting and goal-directed ways.

Functional subgrouping

As I have emphasized, the techniques of functional subgrouping are introduced from the beginning of a systems-centered group. In fact, in new groups, like the inpatient group, defense modification is only used when the techniques of subgrouping are in place. A good example of the difference between the intrapersonal focus of boundarying and the interpersonal focus of subgrouping is that the first step in boundarying requires people to discriminate between their observing self and the experiencing self that they are observing (the distraction exercise will be discussed later in this chapter), whereas the first step in subgrouping (in which people make contact with one another) is put into practice immediately.

> And the first step is to make sure that everybody can see everybody, so, can everybody see everybody without any difficulty?

In systems-centered therapy, all work is done with members either working in functional subgroups or working in relationship to the group-as-a-whole. It is a fundamental technique in SCT groups not to work on the individual member's defenses until the group has some experience of subgrouping so that the working member can experience him or herself working with and for the group and not alone.

The subgrouping doggerel below illustrates how important the use of language is, not only to boundarying, but also in subgrouping, if members are going to be able to subgroup with each other rather than project onto and into each other.

> Asking 'Why are you saying that?'
> or 'Tell me more about that!'
> is like pushing another member's boat out to sea!

> Saying 'I'm in your subgroup'
> is like an encouraging wave from the shore.

> Working as a member of your subgroup
> is more than pushing another member's boat out to sea
> or waving encouragingly from the shore.

> Working in a subgroup
> is getting into a boat and rowing too!

The initial SCT technique for establishing a subgroup is simple. It is basically the phrase 'Anybody else, anybody else!' When there are a lot of 'Yes, buts...' a slightly stronger invitation is useful: 'Please join on a similarity with the last member rather than on your difference – and hold your difference until we have explored what we are working on now.' In groups that have acquired the skills of subgrouping functionally, it is enough to say 'Let's subgroup' or 'There are two sides to this issue in the group – let's subgroup and explore them.'

Making implicit subgroups explicit, another form of functional subgrouping, is more complex and entails identifying the group theme that represents the underlying issue that has salience for the group at that moment. Subgrouping is a conflict resolution technique. If there is no conflict, then members explore group issues together in the group-as-a-whole. If there is conflict, then the SCT therapist identifies the two sides of the conflict in words that are resonant to the group, and asks the group members who is in which of the two subgroups, and which subgroup has the most energy to work first.

The inpatient group script shows how almost my first words draw the group's attention to a common (group-as-a-whole) experience that they can subgroup

[handwritten margin note: Therapist identifies – not the group]

around: 'So the first thing is, how is it for you, in here, on stage, with me, and with people watching, in front of the camera? How is that?'

The group responds with two 'nervous,' one 'exciting,' one 'curious,' one 'guinea pig' and two 'not bothered'. Through the SCT lens I see two potential subgroups: one involved (nervous, excited, curious, and some humor) and one as yet uninvolved (not bothered) (see p.41). Following the hierarchy of defense modification, I start immediately with 'nervous': 'So we have three people who are a little bit anxious about not quite knowing what's going to happen next. Has anybody else joined these three? Anyone else joined since we've been working?' (see p.46)

[handwritten: each member → Monitor my own energy flow / Conscious of when it is directed towards the past/pres/future, reality or unreality, defensive or non-def.]

Boundarying

The purpose of the boundarying techniques is to enable members to direct their *[handwritten: goals]* work energy away from the thoughts that keep their energy out of the group and to deliberately redirect their energy into the group. This requires group members to learn how to monitor their own energy flow, and become conscious when it is directed towards the past, present or future; reality or reality; and towards defensive or non-defensive goals. This is also the technique which SCT calls vectoring, in which members learn to deliberately direct their energy towards their goals (see past/present/future map, Table 3.3, p.119).

The first boundarying techniques to be introduced into a new group are the techniques that govern the way that people bring themselves into a systems-centered group. Boundarying interventions deliberately manage the kinds of communication that cross the boundaries into the group. This is rather like managing pollution of the environment by managing it before it is discharged into the environment. Explicit and implicit punitive super-ego language, for example, with its 'oughts' and 'shoulds' and critical innuendos of self and other are addressed at the boundaries.

In a more experienced group, the major modification work is done at the beginning of each group by the introduction of a simple technique called the 'distraction exercise.' The distraction exercise separates opinions from facts and facts from feelings, so that when the person's feelings enter the group both their communications and their experiences are explicitly related to reality rather than to their fears about reality.

In a beginning group like the inpatient group, however, modifications are managed informally in the process of undoing anxiety and mind-reading and in redirecting social behavior rather than in the distraction exercise.

There are many forms of social behaviors, some of them useful in that they contribute to lightening the atmosphere, others not so useful as they distract a group from its work or tend to monopolize the air time. The social defenses that compete with work are gossip, thinking out loud, story-telling and joking around.

Social behavior is one of the defenses that are modified as soon as they appear, as they are one of the most effective ways to take flight from the here-and-now. Story-telling is a particularly expensive defense on the work that a group has come to do, and SCT modifies it immediately, as was demonstrated in the work with Bill.

Another communication behavior that is modified is the language and thoughts that go with anxiety. All human beings tend to become apprehensive when faced with a new situation, whether it is at the beginning of a group, or at any time they are attempting to communicate something. As was mentioned earlier, SCT frames this as normal 'apprehension at the edge of the unknown,' a form of 'turbulence' at the boundary between the familiar and the unfamiliar that occurs in varying degrees of intensity. When apprehension is contained, it is experienced as potential energy which puts the person in a state of arousal and readiness, ready to explore and discover whatever reality will bring: to explore first and then to explain. When apprehension is not contained, the normal apprehension at the edge of the unknown is experienced as anxiety. When apprehension is transformed into anxiety, the sense of urgency that anxiety generates drives people to explain reality before they explore it, rather than to take the time to explore first and explain second. The human tendency, when anxious, to explain first and explore second is addressed by the SCT technique called 'the fork in the road between explaining and exploring.' Explaining their experience leads people down the road to what they know already about themselves, others and the world. Exploring their experience leads people into exploring and exploring leads into discovering themselves, others and the world. Deliberately choosing to direct their energy into taking one fork or the other is called vectoring energy in SCT.

The way people explain reality is like making a map of the way they see reality. Anxious explanations map an anxious reality which generates negative predictions and still more anxiety. When people believe their anxious maps, the more their emotions are generated by their negative predictions about reality rather than their direct experience of reality. Rather than allowing the negative predictions to govern the behavior that people bring into the group, they are also undone at the boundary with the distraction exercise by the technique called 'the three questions for anxiety.' The three questions for anxiety teach SCT members to become aware that there are three separate sources of anxiety: thoughts, sensations and the experience of apprehension without curiosity, and that they can modify all three through problem-solving and reality testing methods.

They can modify anxiety that comes from thoughts through undoing negative predictions, and checking out their mind-reading and reality testing and by matching their negative predictions. They can modify the anxiety that comes from sensations, feelings and emotions by comparing their thoughts about their experience with their actual experience. SCT members are encouraged to undo the straitjacket of tension that constricts their experience, make space for their internal experience and live in their experience and find out what they know. This is not an easy task.

Context

The major challenge to a SCT therapist in introducing contextualizing is that painful experiences inevitably draw our attention to ourselves, often to the exclusion of anyone or anything else. Requiring group members to pay attention to their context requires them to focus, not only on their personal experience of what is generating their pain, but also on other contexts that exist outside themselves. SCT assumes that much of the pain that brings people into therapy is a matter of personalizing and taking things out of context, that the major work in therapy is not to discover the traumatic incident in the past that will then allow them to live happily ever after in the present. Rather, the work of therapy is to acquire the ability to recognize what prevents one from developing the different, appropriate relationships (roles) to the different contexts that always exist in the here-and-now present.

What is dealt with in any one therapy group and how it is dealt with depends upon two major factors. *What* is dealt with depends upon the phase of development that the group is in. *How* it is dealt with depends upon the specific defenses that are serving as restraints at the boundary.

I have emphasized that the inpatient group, being brand new, was inevitably working in the phase of flight. In other words, there are certain pressures, generic to the first subphase of group development, which all group members experience, and which mobilize flight impulses. SCT assumes that the behavior and experience of an individual member in a group has more to do with the group dynamics than it does with their individual psychodynamics.

Systematically reducing the restraining forces and releasing the driving forces is the fundamental principle of systems-centered practice. Systems-centered leaders enter a new group with a 'map' of the different phases of group development and the specific restraining forces that, when modified, facilitate the development of the group. These restraining forces are sequenced in the SCT hierarchy of defense modification which is separated into five modules, each one of which is relevant to specific issues in a particular phase of development. SCT leaders are careful to reduce only those specific defenses that are relevant to the particular phase that the group is in, so that it is the restraining forces generic to the phase that are modified.

The arousal of flight defenses (intellectualization, vagueness etc.) is not only inherent in the dynamics of the flight phase, it is also predictable. This is what give the technique of defense modification its power. By modifying the flight defenses, in the prescribed order, the members not only do not act out their flight impulses, but they also acquire the skills that will allow them to modify more complex defenses when the phase changes. Flight defenses are not confined to the subphase of flight, nor does the phase of flight preclude other defenses. The entire range of defenses is available whatever the phase of development. Difficulties at any phase of development are likely to arouse constellations of defenses, whether they have already been mastered or not – the greater the difficulty, the more fundamental will be the defense arousal.

Systems-centered work consists of reducing the defenses in a predetermined order (the hierarchy) on the understanding that by following this order, the skills of defense modification build on the skills that have gone before and pave the way for the skills that come next. Thus, work that might have been too difficult if modified prematurely becomes relatively easy to do. This predetermined order is laid out in the SCT Hierarchy of Defense Modification (Agazarian 1999), which synchronizes the particular defense with the particular issues that characterize the developmental phase to which it belongs. This is illustrated in Table 3.2 below.

Table 3.2 The correspondence between the phases of development and the five modules of defense modification

The Hierarchy of Defense Modification in the Context of the Three Phases of Group Development: Authority, Intimacy, Work

Phase One: Hierarchy of defenses against authority

Subphase of flight

Module I.	The social defenses. The triad of symptomatic defenses
Module Ia.	The social defenses: avoidance of unpredictable interpersonal reality by defensive, stereotype, social communications
Module Ib.	The triad of symptomatic defenses
	Cognitive distortions: anxiety-generated maps of reality, based on negative predictions, speculations, worries and other defenses against sitting at the edge of the unknown
	Tension: avoidance of arousal and emotion by tension-generating, stress-related psychosomatic defenses

Transitional phase between flight and fight

Module Ic.	The retaliatory impulse: avoidance of the retaliatory impulse by depression (flight) or hostile acting out of the retaliatory impulse (fight) with targeted or random discharges of irritability, frustration and arousal

Subphase of fight

Module II.	Role locks defenses: defensive projections and projective identifications into one-up/one-down role relationships, like: identified patient/helper; scapegoat/scapegoater; victim/bully; and other defiant/compliant splits that repeat old roles

Transitional phase between authority and intimacy

Module III.   Resistance to change defenses

Externalizing conflicts with authority: defensive stubbornness and suspicion that splits good and bad and blames the bad onto authorities or society from the righteous and complaining position

Disowning authority: defensive stubbornness and suspicion of self that splits good and bad and blames personal incompetence

Phase Two: Hierarchy of defenses against intimacy

Module IV.   Defenses against separation and individuation

Subphase of enchantment and hope

Module IVa.   Defenses against separation: enchantment and blind trust in others, self and groups. Merging and love addiction as a defense against separation

Subphase of disenchantment and despair

Module IVb.   Defenses against individuation: alienation and despair: disenchantment and blind mistrust of self, others and groups

Phase Three: Defenses against interdependent work

Module V.   Defenses against knowing

Module Va.   Defenses against inner reality: defenses against comprehensive and apprehensive knowledge

Module Vb.   Defenses against outer reality: defenses against reality testing in the context of the present realities of role, goal and environment

Below is a brief description of the dynamic issues that are salient to the flight subphase of group development and the specific defenses that SCT modifies in order to contain and explore the dynamics rather than have them acted out in the group.

As I have already mentioned, flight is the phase that is most salient to this chapter as it characterizes the beginning of almost all groups and was certainly characteristic of the inpatient group. This, as you will have seen from the work that the inpatient group did, does not mean that the group spent most of its time in defensive flight. It does mean, however, that the defenses that are deliberately modified in the inpatient unit are the major restraining forces to a group's development into the subsequent phases. As is illustrated in the script, the inpatient group was highly responsive to defense modification and spent a significant amount of time in doing the 'work' that is relevant to the phase of flight. Thus it is not that the flight phase necessarily means that the group is in flight, only that the therapeutic issues that the SCT therapist focuses on are those that are generic to the flight phase.

The defenses that are modified in the flight phase use the techniques of Module I in the hierarchy of defense modification (as shown above in Table 3.2). What follows is a discussion of the course of these modifications in the inpatient group with illustrations taken from the script.

Module I in the hierarchy of defense modification

The first three defenses of Module I are the first of a range of defenses against the kind of energy that is frustration. In Module I the work is to learn how to vector energy: how to focus energy on learning how to work inside one's personal system and literally 'organize it.' Module I work takes the first step towards building system structures that existed only inefficiently before. This is done by training for the basic skills of discrimination that enable boundaries to open and close appropriately, in context, to thoughts and sensations and emotions so that the system is not flooded by undifferentiated emotion (ambiguity) nor brought to a standstill by too much over-discriminated detail (redundancy). This is also done by training for the basics of 'containing' which leads to being able to maintain both sides of a conflict while each side is explored, while the similarities in the apparently different are recognized and the conflict is addressed in reality instead of defended against.

Containing

In SCT, the work of containing is to contain the potential energy until it can be vectored appropriately. Containing potential energy requires containing the frustrating experience of delaying the impulse to act. It is through increasing the capacity to contain that members increase their frustration tolerance and reduce the probability that they will act out.

The major issue in the flight phase is the management of dependency which typically manifests itself in compliance and covert defiance towards the therapist. Each phase has specific differences that are too different to integrate and are therefore split off and projected into a containing group dynamic. In the flight phase, an identified patient role is created to contain the group dependency. The identified patient is offered to the therapist for a cure (unfortunately, over and over again). In systems-centered groups, two containing subgroups split the dependency conflict, one exploring the wish to be taken care of, the other the displacement wish to take care of others instead.

In the inpatient group, Nan was a potential volunteer for the role. As you will see, I responded with the SCT technique of 'keeping her in a box' until she had reconnected with herself, and contained her emotion. Nan had a salience for emotional flooding (we call it a 'deep sea dive' in SCT) and was disappointed that she had not been 'able to open up and spill my feelings.' A flood of emotion is often cathartic for both the group and the member; however, it becomes addictive rather than therapeutic unless the patient learns that her work is to contain emotion so that she can understand it rather than 'spill it' into the group, and unless the group understands that although gratifying, their role of audience is a flight from exploring and understanding their own emotions.

Stereotypic social communication is the first defense to modify in the flight phase. The SCT technique for containing social defenses is the technique of keeping the member in the box. This is often quite hard to do, particularly when members have such an investment in 'telling their story' (over and over again). That this technique was appreciated came in the feedback: 'Her types of meetings wouldn't have wasted as much time as lots of other groups I have been in.'

With the exception of Bill and his leaning towards story-telling, there were very few social defenses in the inpatient group. Bill has the hallmark of a veteran story-teller: 'Well, as I said before, in 1982 I was on the *People are Talking* show with Maury Povitch, I belonged to an organization called Parents without Partners...' (see p.48)

I ask Bill if I may interrupt (trying to put him 'in the box') and he says 'Sure' and I ask him about 'right here-and-now.' With Bill it takes several 'boxing inter-ruptions' and one Mexican stand-off.

> Bill: I am talking about being in the hospital.
>
> Me: Uh, I am talking about being in the group!
>
> Bill: Okay.
>
> Me: Would that be okay if we stayed and focused on the group?
>
> Bill: Yeah, that's fine. The only one thing I wanted to say though...(see p.53)

Bill is a good example of a member who will easily monopolize a group if he is given a chance. In the early stages of this group, I was confident that I could keep him from monopolizing but did not feel very hopeful that we would become attuned to each other, or that he would be able to benefit from the group. One of the best surprises of the group was the work that he did do after his defense was contained, and particularly the insight that he reached: 'I don't feel. I talk *about* my feelings!' So Bill is also a good example of what can happen when one does not enable an entrenched member to use his familiar defenses (nor act out one's own negative predictions).

The response to story-telling in a group is an important part of developing the communication style of the group. From the SCT perspective, all story-telling takes the story-teller, and potentially the group, out of the here-and-now and back into some other place or time.

After social defenses, the major defense modification in the flight phase is the triad of symptomatic defenses. This is the first module of five that define the hierarchy of defense modification. It is called the 'triad of symptomatic defenses' because it addresses the most common symptoms that bring people into therapy: anxiety-provoking thoughts about the future or the present, tension, somatic symptoms and depression.

The triad of symptomatic defenses

The triad of symptomatic defenses addresses three constellations of defense:

1. Cognitive distortions and worrying that divert attention from reality testing.

2. Tension-generating, stress-related psychosomatic defenses, which avoid the experience of emotion.

3. Defending against frustration and the retaliation impulse by constricting it in depression or discharging it in hostile acting out. (This defense modification moves through the transition between the flight and fight subphases.)

In SCT, keeping people connected to both the here-and-now of the group and their conscious, present selves are the primary goals of the first phase of group development. Connecting parallel talk to the underlying group theme becomes important when the group is becoming aware of the group-as-a-whole as a third context for understanding their work. The SCT expectation is that the group theme will surface when the defenses in the group-as-a-whole are sufficiently modified to make it work in a relevant way. The same is true of associations.

There is another extremely important set of techniques for modifying restraining forces at the boundary, and that is the modification of noise in the communication channel. As we know from the discussion of the methods of boundarying, SCT immediately modifies noise with the understanding that the more noise (ambiguities, redundancies and contradictions) in the communication, the less information will be heard. Just like any noise pollution, group energy is diverted into managing the stress that noise causes. Thus, ambiguity or redundancy or contradictions are like an instant alert to a systems-centered therapist.

For example, when I heard Jane respond to my question with 'No, uh, I don't know, haven't given it that much, you know, real thought about it... Yeah, I guess...', the ambiguity flag went up for me. I immediately asked her, 'And is it also for you that it is right on the edge of the unknown?' I'm delighted that Jane managed her own shift into clarity with 'Yes of course,' which I then reinforced: 'So you have just shifted from guess to certainty.'

Anxiety-provoking thoughts, the first defense in the triad

With the inpatient group, undoing anxiety was the first thing to which I turned my attention as soon as I had established a subgroup for the members to work in. Anxiety-provoking thoughts not only make people anxious but also create an imaginary reality that distracts members from their awareness of the reality that exists in the here-and-now of group life. All defense modification is intended to restore the relationship of members to themselves. The triad first reconnects people with their mind, then with their body, then with their emotions.

Modifying anxiety is one of the techniques that puts the method of boundarying into practice. Boundaries are thought about as existing in both real and psychological space and time. In SCT groups, one of the first modifications is to bring to the members' attention that they can time travel in their mind by thinking about the past and the future. This is always all right if the purpose of the trip is to collect information that is useful to the present moment, because then the member is using his or her mind in the service of work. It is not all right when members 'take flight' from the present into the past or the future. It is also an SCT assumption that anxiety has two sources: negative predictions about the future, or negative assumptions about the present. I address the group as follows:

> I want to start, if I may, with 'nervous' – because, very important in this method, is knowing where one's anxieties come from. And sometimes they come from one's thoughts and sometimes they come from one's experience. In terms of being nervous, do you four know whether you were thinking about something that's scaring you? (see pp.42–43)

This is the first of the three questions that SCT uses to undo anxiety, and the first step in teaching these members the technique, with the expectation that if they integrate them, they will be able to ask them of themselves whenever they get anxious. Questions that require members to check their own reality will bring them into their personal present and the present context. The 'three questions for anxiety' are:

1. Are you thinking something that is frightening you? (If so, then the member is asked to identify the anxiety-provoking thought, frequently a negative prediction or a fear of what others are thinking.)

2. Do you have sensations or feelings that are frightening you? (If so, then the member is asked to describe the physical sensations, and to make room for them. In the process, it is usual for members to recognize that the discomfort arose from their attempt to constrict their emotional experience, and when they relax, their experience changes to a pleasant sense of energy. Sometimes the major difference between anxiety and excitement is what we call it!) (see p.42)

3. Are you sitting at the edge of the unknown and feeling anxious about it? (If so, then common reality is affirmed with: 'Everyone is apprehensive at the edge of the unknown and it helps if you can take your curiosity with you.') (see p.42)

The apprehensive response at the edge of the unknown is commonly called anticipatory anxiety. SCT considers anticipatory anxiety a misnomer, in that, when not contaminated by anxiety-provoking thoughts, anticipatory anxiety is a mixture of excitement, alertness, curiosity and a readying of the fight–flight response. SCT assumes that it is containing the frustration of the fight–flight response while the unknown reality is tested, that is defended against by anxiety-provoking thoughts which then generate anxiety. It is for this reason that members are encouraged to mobilize their curiosity about what they will discover at the edge of the unknown. Mobilizing curiosity is a major step towards re-establishing the relationship to reality.

SCT lays great emphasis on framing techniques within a map that connects the technique to the method (in this case boundarying) which in turn relates to the theory (boundaries exist in space and time, contain the group energy and provide the system structure). The frame for boundarying techniques in time is Kurt Lewin's past, present and future, reality and unreality map (Agazarian 1986). The advantage is that it provides a map that makes it quite clear which technique to use when. (see p.119)

Flight into negative predictions (future unreality)

For example, undoing the negative predictions that not only cause anxiety, but also vector members' energy away from the present and into the future, is a simple technique of the three questions that are outlined above. The technical point is that these three questions actually weaken the restraining forces at the boundary and enable the person's energy to return to the present from the future. However, as you will see from the model below, that is only the first boundary to cross. There is still the boundary between unreality and reality. Crossing the first boundary from the future to the present relieves the anxiety, but that is not as important as restoring the connection between the person and whatever impulse, emotion or conflict that they were defending against. Thus, crossing the boundary from present unreality to present reality is the primary goal of defense modification. It makes it easier to keep this in the forefront of one's mind as an SCT therapist if one has access to a mental map.

Table 3.3 Map of the boundaries in space, time and reality (adapted from Lewin 1951 by Yvonne M. Agazarian)

Past, present and future – Experience explained vs. experience explored

	Past	Present	Future
Explaining experience	Interpretations of memory War stories and romances Blaming and complaining	Interpretations based on wishes and fears Thought-generated self-consciousness Criticism of self or other Mind-reading	Negative and positive predictions Anxiety-provoking thoughts Ruminations and worrying Pessimism and optimism about the future
Exploring experience	Past experience Apprehensive memory Emotional intelligence and intuition	Present experience, common sense and reality testing Experience-generated consciousness of self Verbal and emotional intelligence	Plans and goals Curiosity about the unknown Formulating hypotheses Contingency planning

Model illustrating the communication flow across the boundaries from constructed reality into primary reality so that reality testing can take place; external and internal conflicts can be recognized and addressed; and past, present and future reality can be based on primary experience rather than secondary explanation.

Flight into projection (mind-reading)

Mind-reading, the self-consciousness around what others are thinking about you, is another restraining force at the boundary between unreality and reality that calls for a different technique (a different path to the goal). Undoing a mind-read is a more complex event than undoing anxiety. Undoing anxiety requires working with oneself. Undoing mind-reading requires working with another. Typically, it comes later in the group, as it did in the inpatient group. The technique itself is simple but it requires courage of the member to put it into practice. The first step in checking out a mind-read is to ask a 'yes/no' question: a question that someone can answer with a yes or a no. In the interchange with Jane it is clear that it is not as simple as it sounds. I say: 'Would you be willing to check out your assumptions?' Jane says: 'And what, I wouldn't know how.' 'Well, you could ask a question that would get a yes or no answer.' 'Okay, I'll ask, I'll ask a direct question. (*To June*) Are you angry?' (see p.77)

This completes the first step. The second step requires a direct 'yes' or 'no' answer. At this point it is the answering member who is being taught the other side of the technique, which is to take on the role of providing information (to give the data that the questioning member needs in her research). The answering member is encouraged to understand that in the role, nothing is personal – that his or her task is simply to provide the information, and not become personally involved, even though the question is, of course, personal! The SCT techniques are always simple, yet often involve complex learning. In this case, the answering member is learning how to contextualize, to change his or her role appropriate to the context and the goal. This is not easy. For example, June, in answering Jane's question, started to talk about her own experience and I intervened with, 'You are helping Jane to check her reality, and what you are doing is you are telling Jane that the way she thinks and the way you are, are two different things... You are doing some pretty important work.' I then ask, 'Do you believe her, Jane?' (see p.78)

This is an important third step for both the member and the group. It starts the process of legitimizing reality testing in the group and it requires the person who is checking reality to pay attention to their own process of validation. If they say no, the next question is 'What is it like for you to work in a group knowing that there is a member in it that you don't trust to tell you the truth?' This, as you can see, is an even more important step in bringing both the member and the group into reality, and includes in the focus both the trust issue and also trust as it relates to the realities of work.

The third step asks the question 'How does it feel to have your reality confirmed (or denied)?' Again, the greater learning comes from the difference. When the reality is denied the member has an opportunity to recognize his or her particular reactions to cognitive dissonance.

The importance of this is well illustrated in the following dialogue. Incidently, this is the Jane of the flaccid hands who did not appear, at the beginning of the group, as a likely candidate for the courageous kind of work she did here.

> YA: So you don't believe that June isn't angry right now, even though she has told you that she isn't?
>
> Jane: Right.
>
> YA: So how is that for you – to check your reality and find out that June has a different reality from yours? And that you don't believe her?
>
> Jane: Mmm.
>
> YA: How does that feel?

Jane: Well, I feel as though, uh, you know that I have to rethink, but, uh, at the same time my first, uh, my first impression, uh, you know, already said yes…

YA: So it is hard to change your mind is it?

Jane: Well not at the moment.

YA: Yes. Is that one of the difficulties you have?

Jane: Yeah.

YA: Okay, so now we have for you, in this group, one of the same kinds of difficulties that you have outside?

Jane: Mmm.

YA: Okay?

Jane: I guess so.

YA: You guess so or it is true?

Jane: Well, I'll have to say it is true. I totally agree. (see p.78)

Flight into the past

Modifying the restraining force at the boundary between the past and the present is another simple technique. There is first an important discrimination to be made. Is going to the past a flight from the present? Or is it in the service of getting information that is useful in managing the challenges of the present? Much wasted time in therapy is avoided if this discrimination is made. Modifying the restraining force at the boundary between the past and the present is even simpler than modifying the boundary between the present and the future. The technique is simply a matter of changing a word or two. To vector a person's energy from the past to the present one simply asks 'How is the present different from the past?' The reverse is also true; to vector energy back to the past one asks 'How is the present similar to your past?' The past to present question is easy to ask; how powerful it is, is easily understood when one sees how difficult it is sometimes for people to see the differences between the past and the present, even when they are quite obvious. We are of course talking of transference, which in SCT is neutralized in the beginning stages of therapy by making the distortions conscious, and dealt with only when earlier defenses against it are modified and the role-lock and pervasive transferences are next in the hierarchy (Agazarian 1994). The most subtle form of flight into the past sounds as if the member is joining with another member, or joining a subgroup, when in reality they are not.

Bill: If you had spoken to me three days ago I would have had a feeling of anger. (see p.76)

The fork in the road between explain and explore is, of course, always available as a technique for encouraging people across the past to present boundaries.

> YA: (*To Josh*) Okay, so what I'd like to say to you also, if you go outside and back into your past and match what's happening now with what's happened before, you may come up with a good *explanation*, but what you would miss is anything new you discover from living in the here-and-now. If you *explore* the experience, and wait and work in the group, you may just discover that there is something that you didn't know about yourself. (see p.59)

The explore–explain dichotomy is one of the most important that is addressed in SCT for the very reasons that I submitted to Josh. The explore–explain conflict lies at the boundary between secondary and primary reality, and is one of the easiest restraining forces to weaken. In systems-centered groups members are interrupted if they explain, and it is pointed out to them that explaining takes them into the world they know already, whereas exploring takes them into their experience and into the unknown.

Below is another version of the explore–explain fork in the road as illustrated in a force field contrasting the driving and restraining forces between working in the here-and-now and taking flight into the past or present.

Table 3.4 Force field of driving and restraining forces in relationship to the here-and-now, past or present	
Driving forces →	← *Restraining forces*
Explore →	← Explain
Checking out whether someone is thinking what you think they think →	← Mind-reading
Collecting data about what you know about the future →	← Negative predictions
Discriminating between the present and the past →	Failing to discriminate between the ← present and the past

In SCT work, there is always a deliberate redirection of energy away from the past or the future and into the present. This brings members sufficiently into the here-and-now for group reality to be sufficiently consciously shared and lived in.

Equally important is the SCT understanding that the people who are in a group only become members of a group when they are present in it. When they leave the group and go into their personal roles in the past, present or future, they are no longer in their member role in the group. When people psychologically 'leave the group,' whatever here-and-now conflict triggered the flight is not in focus, and is often unnoticed and unconnected to the defensive maneuver. SCT understands the associative process to serve primarily as a defense, in which members manage stressors in the present by retreating to a look-alike in the past. This avoids the fear of pain in the present. But it also transfers the person back into a previous time of remembered pain, which, though it has the advantage of relieving the uncertainty of the moment, replaces the pain of uncertainty in the present with the pain of the past. An important principle in SCT is to encourage the members to contrast their familiar failures with the unknown potentials for failure in the group, and discover which feels worst.

Flight to the past confronts members with another fork in the road between whatever the conflict is in the present that is being avoided by a retreat to a 'look-alike' in the past.

Keeping the member in the box

Keeping the member in the box is the technique of following them wherever they go, undoing whatever phase-appropriate defense that takes them away from the task of exploring the realities of themselves, others and their environment. Small examples of 'boxing' are my questions that change a speculation ('Maybe, perhaps, I think so') into a committed statement like "yes", or "no", or "I do". Keeping members in a box requires being sufficiently attuned to have a sense when they have taken flight so that you can call them back and hold them to their work. Sometimes the pay-off is very rewarding, and other times it is very sad. The first example pays off for Nan. The second example is poignant, and it may pay off or it may not.

> YA: (*To Nan*) You said you were scared? I am going to ask you the same question, which is, are you thinking something that is frightening you?
>
> Nan: Yes.
>
> YA: What are you thinking?
>
> Nan: Oh boy! I am really scared now.
>
> YA: Well, you know, thoughts that are inside one's head...
>
> Nan: Mmm... (*Nan nods like an obedient child.*)
>
> YA: ...are always more frightening than after you have said them.
>
> Nan: Okay. That's true.

YA: So, would you test that out?

Nan: Okay, I will. (*Nan takes a deep breath and looks up to the ceiling.*) I have a way of covering up my feelings with my family…

YA: Okay. Right this moment, you said you were scared…

Nan: Yeah. It's, it's, let me just… (*holds up a finger to stop me*)

YA: (*I interrupt*) Is there anything at all that you are thinking?

Nan: Yeah (*her finger goes up again*).

YA: …about this group?

Nan: Yes (*finger goes up*).

YA: What?

Nan: Just a few minutes ago (*she holds her finger up high as if pointing*), just a few minutes ago I went outside and met my dad.

YA: Uh-huh.

Nan: And it frightened me.

YA: Okay. So you went outside and you *thought* about your dad?

Nan: I thought about him and I got all upset, and my stomach started turning.

YA: Was that while you were in this group?

Nan: It was right before I came to this group.

YA: How about since you've been in this group? Has anything happened?

Nan: I feel more calmer.

YA: You do?

Nan: Mmm.

YA: So is there anything that is frightening you right now?

Nan: Uh. (*This time Nan stays in eye contact, appears calm and appears to be checking with herself.*)

YA: Do you feel frightened right now?

Nan: No! (*She shakes her head with assurance. She is no longer showing any signs of agitation.*) (see pp.55–56)

In the above example, keeping Nan in the box resulted in her being able to come into the reality that here-and-now was okay, whereas her imagined reality was not. It is also an excellent example of how easily the gratification of the drama of imagined reality competes and wins over the actual demands of here-and-now reality.

The work below is a crucial piece of work for Al. Earlier in the group I had asked Al 'If you had a completely free choice, which would you rather do – stay in the group or go out and worry?' (p.58) and Al had answered immediately 'Stay in the group.' In the work below, he too breaks through to his inner experience, but with a different affect from Nan's. This is a serious example of how, when a member confronts the costs and costs of a defense, the costs sometimes outweigh the benefits. This introduces the therapeutic issue of making the defense sufficiently ego-dystonic to make it worthwhile to explore the alternative.

YA: So right this moment...I think you just went on to automatic there and answered the question the way you've answered it before rather than checking with your experience right here-and-now. Is that right? (see p.81)

Al: Yeah.

YA: Okay, so if you check with your experience about being in this group and sitting on the fence and paying attention and noticing that you felt curious and aroused, you noticed your experience then – and noticing that part of you had to compete with the part of you that is pulling you apart...

Al: I don't know.

YA: In this last half-hour has it been worth it or has it not?

Al: No, it hasn't been worth it.

YA: It hasn't been worth it.

Al: Not really.

YA: It hasn't been worth it?

Al: Not really.

YA: How do you feel about that, that somehow...

Al: I didn't...

YA: If you would...

Al: I have never had much experience.

YA: Take your time, take your time because if you answer too soon you're not going to notice how you feel. Do you understand me?

Al: It's all blocked up.

YA: Wait! Whoa! If you answer too soon, you are not going to notice how you feel. Do you want to know how you feel? It's up to you (*pause*), it really is up to you right this moment.

Al: Yes.

YA: You want to?

Al: Yes.

YA: Okay, so how do you feel?

Al: Sad. (see pp.82–83)

This is the moment when the world stands still.

Tension, the second defense in the triad

When anxiety is reduced in a group, the next defense expected is the defense of tension. Tension also occurred in this group, but it was too early in the process to undo. The group has not yet learned the fork in the road, and therefore does not know that with every defense there is something that is being defended against – in other words, the requisite skill level has not been reached, either of defense modification or subgrouping. The SCT frame for tension is: tension is a strait-jacket that constricts the experience of emotion.

Josh says 'Physically I am a little tense or becoming tense' and I take the opportunity to introduce tension: 'One of the ways that we think about tension is that we sort of clamp down on our body and stop ourselves from having feelings.' (see p.46)

The SCT technique for undoing tension is to ask the member either to let it drain away, or to go and live inside the tension and see what he or she discovers. It is a matter of surprise how often framing tension as a straitjacket for feeling and suggesting that the person undo it succeeds. When it doesn't, we use the bracketing technique, which we also use for undoing somatic symptoms and depression when they occur in a group. There is an important distinction to be made between defenses that are related to responses in the group (like tension, or a sudden headache) and defenses that are so habitual that they have become part of the character structure. Character defenses are not addressed until after the fight–flight phase when the group is working with undoing 'role locks.' In the bracketing technique a 'bracket' is put around what was going on in the group when the member first noticed the headache, for example, and what was going on in the group before they had a headache. A step by microstep of the events between 'no headache' and 'headache' typically surfaces a reaction that they had considered unacceptable. Typically, with the recognition, the symptoms vanish (Agazarian 1997).

Turning the researcher on

I am not going to address Josh's tension at this time in the group in that I have only introduced the first steps in the modification of anxiety.[6] Instead, I try to mobilize Josh's curiosity about himself.

Josh is cautious, with a strong intellectualizing defense. Enlisting the part of Josh that could eventually enable him to access his emotional intelligence is a good alternative. 'Are you curious about why you are tense?' I ask him. 'Yeah, actually I am,' he says. 'Okay. So we don't know at the moment. It may be that you are having a feeling that you don't know about.' 'Maybe.' 'Or it may be something else. We will just have to wait and see.' (see p.47)

Techniques for beginning and ending an SCT group

There are two important SCT techniques that we have only mentioned in passing, one at the beginning and the other at the end of each group meeting. The beginning technique is called the distraction exercise, and is established as soon as the norms of the group have been established. The distraction exercise is a technique for bringing people across both psychological and temporal bound- aries so that they can vector their energy into the here-and-now of the group. This technique is not brought into the group until after the group has the support of subgrouping, and after the individual work at the boundary is recognized as work for the group as well as for the member who is doing the work. The ending technique called 'Suprises and Learnings' is discussed below (see p.129).

The distraction exercise

Like so many of the techniques in SCT, the technique of the distraction exercise comprises a series of reality-testing questions. The first question is to the group: 'Does anyone have a distraction that is keeping their working energy out of the group?' If a member says yes, they are asked to state their distraction, 'Facts first, feelings second.'

There are three important dynamics involved in the distraction exercise. First of all it requires members to discriminate between the world of facts and the world of feelings. This is the first step in orienting the member to the SCT goal which is to discriminate between comprehensive and apprehensive knowledge, and acquire the skill of making the boundary permeable between the two kinds of knowledge so that intuitive understanding can be integrated verbally and vice versa. This is also a primary discrimination, the first discrimination that SCT members explicitly make that begins to establish their 'researcher'.[7]

Second, if feelings come first, there is no way of knowing whether they are being generated by thoughts or whether they are being generated by emotional experience. This is a fundamental discrimination in SCT.

As we have discussed previously in this chapter, in SCT, feelings are not synonymous with emotion. Emotion is essentially a nonverbal *experience*. Emotions are communicated through nonverbal intention movements. Emotions must be translated into feelings before they can be communicated verbally. In the distraction exercise, for example, if someone makes a fist without knowing it, the leader will ask 'What's in your hand?' If the person still doesn't know (we discourage guessing) then the leader will say 'So your body knows something you don't yet know!' In contrast, when feelings serve as a direct translation of emotion, then the person is engaged in the process of discriminating and integrating their experience: sometimes discovering new emotional depths in themselves, sometimes gaining emotional insight, sometimes finding words to fit their experience.

SCT lays great emphasis on subgrouping to explore rather than defend against or act out emotional 'intentions,' making the assumption that translating emotions helps contain them. A good example of how translating emotional impulse into words helps contain it comes from a story about the little chimp Lucy, who loved being tickled, and would rush at her trainer for a tickle. As she got bigger, her enthusiastic 'tickle' impulse threatened to overwhelm her trainer. When the trainer would sign to Lucy 'What does Lucy want?', Lucy would pause and sign back 'Tickle.' Each time the trainer and Lucy communicated, Lucy's enthusiasm became more contained, and her trainer was in less danger of being bowled over.

It is this same dynamic, filtering an emotional impulse through communication (which involves cognition and comprehension), that enables SCT groups to explore the familiar impulses rather than acting them out. And training starts with the distraction exercise.[7]

The technique of the distraction exercise is a series of questions (the therapist's) and answers (the patient's). In our groups for patients for whom human contact is at least as important as learning the skills to manage their conflicts, the question is changed to 'distractions or news.' It then gives them an opportunity to report the good and bad of the week, and keep each other up to date.

One question would be: 'Do you have a distraction that is keeping your energy out of the group?' If the answer is yes, the therapist might ask: 'Will you please separate the facts of your distraction from your feelings about it?' This gives the therapist an opportunity to teach the patient to be specific, succinct and relevant about what is distracting them. Many patients experience great relief as they make the separation between opinion, facts and feelings.

'How do you feel about those facts?' This gives the therapist the opportunity to teach the patient to discriminate between feelings that are in direct response to the described event, and feelings that are generated from the frame that they have used to interpret the event.

'Will you please leave the facts outside the group and bring your feelings into the group by making silent eye contact with each member and bring your feeling into your relationship with them?' This establishes pairing in the service of work, and lays the groundwork for attunement, resonance and future subgrouping. It also gives the 'distracted' member practice in bringing their feelings into a relationship, and gives the 'receiving' member practice in not taking someone else's feelings personally. It makes an invaluable contribution to the transition between flight and fight, and does much to undo the fear that people easily have when someone is frustrated or angry.

Surprises, learning, satisfactions, dissatisfactions and discoveries

As you will see from the following script, this is an important transition out of the group which gives the members the opportunity to review their work, to relate it to their goals, and to frame their satisfactions and dissatisfactions in terms of the driving and restraining forces in a force field. Surprises are the 'differences' that the members were not expecting and which give them an opportunity to integrate experience in a new way. Learning is the cognitive understanding they may have come to. And discoveries are the intuitive experience that often come in the form of insight.

With Bill I introduce the idea that a disappointment can be a guide for next steps in work: 'The useful thing about disappointment is to see what you could do so that you don't get so disappointed again. So can you think of one thing that you did in here this afternoon that made it harder for you to bring your feelings in, which is what you want to do, one thing that you would be able to change in a half hour?' (*Bill shrugs.*) 'If you shrug you're not going to be really engaged in the conflict and find out what is the one thing that you did in here this afternoon which if you *don't do* in a half hour you have a better chance of bringing your feelings in, which is what you want to do.' It is in this transition that Bill gets his insight (see pp.87–89):

Bill: I don't...

YA: Yes you do, so let's hang in there. What would be one thing you could do differently in the group in a half hour so that you have a better chance of doing what you want to do, which is to bring your feelings in?

Bill: Yes. Just be honest.

YA: And so what would you do honestly in a half hour in the group that you didn't do in here?

Bill: I'd talk about my feelings, I would feel...

YA: As you are talking?

Bill: As I'm talking.

YA: Yes, okay.

Bill: I don't feel, I talk *about* my feelings.

YA: (*To Rose*) Do you know one thing that you did today that took you in the direction that you want to go, that you would want to do more of?

Rose: Even more focusing on...focusing on right now.

Sam: That's the main thing, to hell with the next hour and a half. (*Gestures 'right here.'*)

YA: Right, 'cause the moment that we're living is right now, isn't it?

You can't win them all – not all the goal formulations turn out as I would wish! There's no clear feedback from Al: 'Are you on the fence? Or have you dropped out?' Al says, 'Mostly, on.'

Nan says, 'I'm disappointed in myself.' I respond: 'Well let's see if we can turn that disappointment into your next step. What would you like to have done here that you didn't?' 'Open up and be able to spill my feelings.'

Josh is also disappointed: 'Well, I've got a glimpse of the state that you're trying to get us to reach and a couple of the people have said they did reach and I'm not sure what your purpose is but I see a value in it and it's as you said, but I'm not able so far to get anywhere, and it feels good.'

YA: So, did you notice any things that you did today that may have slowed you up?

Josh: It's hard to say because I'm trying so to go to a certain place and I can't see what direction it is – and I'm searching in all directions for explanations, methods, whatever, but I don't see anything useful.

YA: Okay, so what I would say is that there's always a fork in the road between explaining things and exploring things.

Josh: I couldn't see it, don't see that.

YA: Yes, I understand that. But maybe when you have the opportunity, when it feels right for you, if you would hold the explanations aside for awhile and just see what you discover instead, at some time when it feels right for you, you try that. Explore your experience instead of explaining it. And maybe you can get help to learn how to do that. (see p.92)

Conclusion

The inpatient group was a brand new group. For brand new groups in SCT the first few sessions are predominantly a teaching and learning experience. New ways of thinking and speaking are introduced that differentiates the systems-centered group experience from the more traditional psychodynamic approaches. In systems-centered groups, members are required to discover the reality of unconscious and conscious experience through exploration without interpretation. For systems-centered therapy to work, the descriptive, depathologizing understanding of dynamics common to all living human systems must be put in place before the major dynamic issues of therapy are addressed.

This means putting into practice the systems-centered techniques that make the theory and its methods real in the experience of the members of the group.

All systems-centered work is viewed in context. The different phases of system development serve as different contexts, each one of which contains a phase-appropriate set of goals; each one of which has specific requirements for phase-appropriate defense modification; and each one of which is in itself a step in a hierarchical sequence that increases the ability to survive, develop and transform.

This shaping of behavior occurs from the first few seconds the group puts into practice the basic SCT understanding of change. The SCT change hypothesis suggests that the driving force in living human systems is spontaneously vectored towards the goals of survival, development and transformation. SCT understands the dynamics of change to operate like a force field, in which the location of the system on the path to the goals can be explained, at any point in time, as the result of the driving forces towards the goal, and the restraining forces away from the goal.

'Living' in their experience instead of thinking or talking about it is the introduction to the two routes to knowledge that are accessed in SCT: *comprehension* and *apprehension*. Comprehensive knowledge comes from man's imaginative conceptualizations of reality. Words come first and understanding second. Apprehensive knowledge comes from intuitions about reality: understanding comes first and words second. It sometimes takes man years to put into words what he understood intuitively in an instant. Making the boundary permeable between comprehension and the world of understanding based on testing reality, making cognitive maps of the way to man's goals and solving the problems that lie in the way, and experiencing the curiosity that is only assuaged through an apprehensive world of understanding that is older than man, *is* the goal of systems-centered therapy.

For those interested in theory, the force field depicts two goal relationships – the system driving forces are the natural life forces, and the restraining forces are the forces of defense. The driving forces represent energy in the mass/energy equation, and the restraining forces represent mass. Driving forces serve a change function and restraining forces serve a system maintenance function.

Notes

1   The method of functional subgrouping tests the assumption that systems survive, develop and transform from simpler to more complex through the process of discriminating and integrating differences.

2   Agazarian and Simon (Simon and Agazarian 1967; Simon and Agazarian 2000) developed a behavioral system called SAVI (System for Analyzing Information) that assesses the problem-solving potential in any communication (group or individual) by determining the balance between noisy and clear language.

3   Theoretically, it is assumed that emotions carry apprehensive information and are the source of emotional intelligence, that feelings are comprehensive and one of the sources that humans use to make their cognitive maps. The cognitive skills for map-making are measured by IQ (verbal intelligence), and the ability to have and translate emotional experience into common sense responses is EQ (emotional intelligence) (Goleman 1995).

4   SCT places much importance in therapist training on this tendency to split good and bad when the going gets rough. For example, in supervision, there is much emphasis on how therapists have a tendency to diagnose a patient when they are frustrated with them – thus giving them the 'bad patient' label and keeping themselves as 'good.' This can rebound, of course, and then the therapist too becomes 'bad.' Supervision is reframed for the SCT therapist. The presentation starts not with what the supervisee thinks the patient's problem is, but what the supervisee's problem is.

5   The language of rowing is the subjective 'I,' not the accusative 'you.'

6   If there was the possibility of continuing with this group, I would expect, from the level of work that is being done in their first session, that it would be possible to address tension, other psychosomatic symptoms and the postures that reinforce maladaptive roles, in the second or third session.

7   The 'researcher' is the practical manifestation of the observing system, which develops the ability to discriminate and integrate differences. The 'researcher' is developed in members in the initial phases of group: on the one hand establishing a reality testing climate in the group, and on the other hand reducing the restraining forces, in the individuals, to testing the realities of the here-and-now. The 'researcher' in members enables them to cross the boundaries in time: from dread of the future to testing the reality of the negative predictions in the present, from importing the past into the present by observing how the present is different from the past, and from present concerns about what others are thinking by checking out whether or not others are thinking what they 'think' they are thinking.

Members are initially introduced to how to undo their anxieties by discovering the fork in the road between the defense and whatever impulse, conflict or reality experience that they are defending against. The 'fork in the road' technique holds as a reliable method for undoing the increasingly complex defenses in the hierarchy of defense modification, and brings members into a useful and satisfying relationship to their apprehensive and comprehensive understandings.

CHAPTER FOUR

The Theory behind the Practice of Systems-Centered Therapy

A theory of living human systems defines a hierarchy of isomorphic systems that are energy-organizing, goal-directed and self-correcting (Agazarian 1997, see the chart on p.134).

Thinking systems

The single most important thing to remember when we are theorizing about systems is that a theory is a set of ideas that have no reality except in the mind. For those who like to play with ideas, developing theory is a compelling activity which is sometimes unbearably frustrating and at others extraordinarily satisfying. Exciting too, when one becomes curious as to whether or not the new ideas that develop as the theory develops will lead to discovering something one didn't know about the real world. This is the transition between the theorizing and translating theory into practice.

It has been, and continues to be, my ambition to define the constructs of theory clearly enough so that a clear connection can be drawn from the constructs to the methods that are developed from the constructs and in turn the techniques that put these methods into practice. Systems-centered therapy was developed from a theory of living human systems (Agazarian 1997). If systems-centered therapy does indeed serve as a blueprint for treatment that can reliably predict where a patient is in their therapy by assessing where they are in the hierarchy of defense modification, and if the sequence of defense modification does correlate reliably with a reduction in the symptoms that is predicted through the modification of each defense, then a theory of living human systems will have been validated and its methods demonstrated to be reliable. In the service of this task, it continues to be my ambition that each SCT intervention serves as a testable

A THEORY OF LIVING HUMAN SYSTEMS AND ITS SYSTEMS-CENTERED® PRACTICE
Yvonne M. Agazarian
A theory of living human systems defines a hierarchy of isomorphic
systems that are energy-organizing, self-correcting and goal-directed.

THEORETICAL DEFINITIONS

HIERARCHY	ISOMORPHY		
Every system exists in the environment of the system above and is the environment for the system below.	Systems are similar in structure and function and different in different contexts. There is an interdependent relationship between the dynamics of structure, function and energy.		
	Structure	**Energy**	**Function**
System-centered hierarchy The systems-centered hierarchy is defined by the member system, the subgroup system and the group-as-a-whole system	systems-centered structure define boundaries in space, time and reality that are potentially permeable to information.	systems-centered energy/ information is defined as a force field of vectors approaching or avoiding system goals.	systems-centered systems function to survive, develop and transform by discriminating and integrating information.

SYSTEMS-CENTERED METHODS

contextualizing: developing the systems-centered hierarchy.	**Boundarying:** organizing energy / information.	**Vectoring:** directing energy / information.	**Subgrouping:** correcting energy / information.
Person system: primary personality **Observing self-system:** discriminates & integrates information. **Member system:** directs energy into sub-groups. **Subgroup system:** contains and explores information. **Group-as-a-whole system** integrates information.	Survival: managing the permeability of system boundaries (in the hierarchy of systems) by reducing noise in the communications within and between systems.	Development: directing information towards the primary goals of survival, development and transformation and/or towards the secondary environmental task goals.	Transformation: containing, discriminating and integrating differences (in similarity) and similarities (in difference) at all three system levels.

SYSTEMS-CENTERED TECHNIQUES

Eliciting the SCT group requires developing an observing self-system and establishing the member, subgroup and group-as-a-whole roles by using boundarying, subgrouping and vectoring interventions tailored to the context of each phase of system development.	Applying the SCT "Hierarchy of Defense Modification" weakens the restraining forces to valid communication and releases the drive towards system goals.	The "fork-in-the-road" techniques frees the energy bound up in defenses and redirects it towards exploring the conflicts or impulses defended against.	The SCT conflict-resolution technique of "Functional Subgrouping" contains, explores and integrates differences instead of stereotyping or scapegoating them.

Figure 4.1 The Theory of Living Systems (TLHS) and its Systems-Centered Practice (SCT). The theory of living human systems defines a hierarchy of isomorphic systems that are energy organizing, self-correcting and goal directed.

hypothesis so that the therapist can get immediate feedback as to how reliably the therapeutic system is traveling along the path to the therapeutic goals. To this end, this chapter contains descriptive statements of the theory, and its constructs and their connection to the methods and techniques of systems-centered practice.

A theory of living human systems

Von Bertalanffy (1969) states that every living system is essentially an open system. It maintains itself in a continuous inflow and outflow. A system is closed if nothing enters or leaves. It is open if there is a continuous exchange of matter and energy. In fact, this process of energy and material transformations in cells is the very essence of life. The concepts within von Bertalanffy's general systems theory, such as isomorphy, hierarchy, boundary permeability, energy, goals, and transformation, are all the building blocks that I have used to develop a theory of living human systems.

In developing a theory of living human systems, I have contributed to the work of theorizing with a defined set of constructs that relate one to another and, most important of all, a set of definitions that has generated a real world practice in systems-centered therapy.

There were several steps in this process. The first was to formulate the statement 'a theory of living human systems defines a hierarchy of isomorphic systems that are energy-organizing, self-correcting and goal-directed.' Next, I had to find a definition for each one of the words that constructed the statement. As this was still the world of theory, I was happy and absorbed in the task. Next came the challenge of building the bridge between the world of ideas and the real world of practice. Each theoretical definition required reformulating so that it could be applied in reality. In other words, each required an operational definition from which hypotheses could be generated and tested. The operational definition that I formulated for a theory of living human systems became the methods of contextualizing, boundarying, subgrouping and vectoring, which were the methods which would bring into reality a systems-centered group. The last step was to test the validity of the theory and the reliability of its practice. As the theory was tested in reality over time, techniques were developed that reliably put the methods into practice which then enabled SCT therapists to test whether an SCT group changes in the directions predicted.

A theory of living human systems defines a hierarchy of isomorphic systems that are energy-organizing, self-correcting and goal-directed (Agazarian 1997). Structurally, each system in the hierarchy is defined by its boundaries; functionally, systems survive, develop and transform through splitting, containing and integrating differences. Boundarying, subgrouping, vectoring and contextualizing are introduced as methods which develop the systems-centered group in which people learn to become systems-centered rather than self-centered.

Definition of hierarchy

The first construct in the theory to be defined is hierarchy. Every system in a defined hierarchy of systems exists in the environment of the system above it and is the environment for the system below it. The hierarchy defined for all living human systems is the system of member, subsystem and system-as-a-whole.

Using systems language solved a problem that I had been wrestling with for 30 years: how to think about the group without having to think about the individual members in terms of their psychodynamics and the group in terms of its group dynamics. Systems theory had provided a set of common concepts to think about the individual and the group as systems. The definition of hierarchy enabled me to use a common language to describe the dynamics of individuals and groups (Agazarian 1993).

In earlier attempts to solve the problem I had postulated 'role' as a bridge between the individual and the group (Agazarian 1982; Agazarian and Peters 1981). Just as the person had characteristic roles that he or she played out in the group, so the group had characteristic roles, like the identified patient or scapegoat, that it played out in the group. The power of group therapy is that many volunteer for these roles in the group but few are chosen.

With this systems definition of hierarchy there was no longer a need for a bridge construct. The person-as-a-whole took up membership in an internal subgroup, and joined the look-alike subgroup in the group. Another important outcome of defining hierarchy was that it added an additional level of abstraction. SCT introduced the idea of 'subgroup' to group psychotherapy as an idea as important as the ideas of member and group. We are used to reifying ideas, and it is often difficult to remember that the system of group is not the group itself, nor is the system of member and subgroup. They come into existence as ideas in the mind, and they are not more than passing imaginations unless we can do something in the real world with real members and subgroups and groups that we could not do before we had those ideas. Introducing three levels of abstraction had great significance. It led to the development of functional subgrouping as a conflict resolution technique – and most important of all, it provided a way of thinking and doing that brought into reality the systems-centered group.

Method of contextualizing

In systems-centered therapy, hierarchy is operationalized by the method called contextualizing by which the observing self-system and the role functions of member, subgroup and group-as-a-whole are developed.

The importance of contextualizing is that it develops the systems-centered frame which, when members understand it, enables them to do what they could not do before they understood it. They are able to recognize that taking things personally belongs to a different way of thinking than taking things in context.[1]

Developing the concepts of member, subgroup and group-as-a-whole is like drawing a conceptual map. Once it exists as a map, it can serve as predictor of behavior for those who have access to the map and want to use it. The advantage of the contextualized map is that it is the same map for all members of a systems-centered group, although each member may be at a different stage of drawing it or using it.

The techniques chapter (Chapter Three) discusses the cost of misconstructed maps, and the techniques that SCT uses to undo the cognitive distortions and other defenses by learning to become a researcher. Contextualizing is not about undoing misconstructions, nor about becoming a researcher, it is about developing a mental construction in the mind of the people in the group – a construction of the member, the subgroup and the group-as-a-whole.

Learning to see things from these different contexts enables members to recognize that their communications have a meaning, not only for themselves, and not only for their subgroup, but also for the group-as-a-whole. As they see this they discover their experience shifts as the context shifts. It is thus that they learn to hear themselves give voice for their person system and three other systems (member, subgroup and group-as-a-whole). It is through understanding the context of their experience that members learn not to take things 'just' personally.

The methods of contextualizing are not intuitively obvious, like the methods of boundarying, subgrouping and vectoring. It is a way of thinking that has to be learned, and the learning is done as part of a developmental process. For example, the first step in the learning is to recognize the difference between being self-centered and systems-centered. As self-centered, the self is the only context. SCT calls this a barrier experience (Agazarian 1997), because the boundaries are permeable only to information that confirms perception. As systems-centered, the person is aware of both the context of the self and the context of the environment. In contextualizing, those 'environments' are specifically the systems of member, subgroup and group-as-a-whole.

The first step in this process is to develop what SCT calls an observing system whose function is to discriminate and integrate information about reality.[2] This is done immediately and simply in SCT by drawing members' attention to the difference between thinking and emotion. The distraction exercise at the initial boundarying into each group session introduces the first formal learning step. The informal training is the continuing pressure to recognize the fork in the road between exploring experience and explaining it. The second step in the fork in the road is to discover what was being defended against, and this leads to the unknown and apprehensive experience. A major goal in SCT is to make the boundary appropriately permeable between apprehension and comprehension.

In the process of developing their observing self-system, people acquire the ability to experience themselves, not only as a person-as-a-whole with membership in many internal subgroups (a functional self-centered system) but also as members of the group-as-a-whole and its subgroups. Contextualizing involves developing an awareness of the self in the role that is appropriate to the context – which has as many emotional meanings as there are contexts to understand it from.

Definition of isomorphy

The theoretical definition of isomorphy is that systems are similar in structure and function and different in different contexts. The systems of member, subgroup and the group-as-a-whole are similar in structure, function and dynamic principles of operation.

The system definition of isomorphy introduces an important functional difference. It is the difference between thinking like Aristotle, who said that whatever one says a thing is, then it is – a chair is a chair is a chair; and Korzybski, who said whatever one says a thing is, it is not – a chair is a chair is a table, is a step ladder, is a bookcase, is a clothes horse. All it takes is a shift in the frame of reference (Agazarian 1992; Korzybski 1948).

Functional thinking effectively disposes of the problem of whether a group-as-a-whole 'is really' just a collection of individuals, or whether it 'is really' something quite different. It is of course always both. What it 'is' at any one time will depend upon the purpose for which it is being described – the perspective from which it is useful to the 'thinker' to 'think.'

Thinking of 'individual,' 'subgroup' and 'group' as three 'systems' in a hierarchy of related systems requires an additional discipline of thinking, but one which does not contradict the existing body of psychodynamic knowledge. In fact, SCT draws heavily upon psychodynamics when it comes to the application of the theory in practice. A systems perspective, however, does provide an additional way of looking at the dynamics of both the individual and the group, so that the combined understanding of group and individual dynamics can be applied to the practice of group psychotherapy. The additional dimension that systems thinking introduces is complementarity.

Complementarity is a basic orientation in systems thinking (Agazarian and Janoff 1993). Like yin/yang, it describes the principle of always being separate, yet always related. In SCT, dynamics are thought about in terms of either/or *only* when dichotomizing is useful.

Because systems in a hierarchy are isomorphic, what one learns about any one level of experience can be applied to any other level. Thus not only is it possible to learn more about the world of group in all three dimensions, but also about oneself. (A great motivator to learn not to take things 'just' personally.)

Structure and function[3]

Structure and function are the constructs that define the isomorphy of systems in the hierarchy.[4] Structure is determined by the system boundaries in space and time. Boundary permeability determines what information enters or leaves the system. Function determines how the information is processed. Function is determined by the principles by which the system operates.

Systems develop by making their boundaries appropriately permeable to the communications that occur between systems, among systems and within systems in the hierarchy. Systems open their boundaries to information that is similar enough to be integrated and close them to information that is too different.

Systems close boundaries to differences that are too different. Systems have difficulty with differences. Differences introduce new information into the system and before the system can integrate it, the new information has to be organized, and the existing organization has to be reorganized.

There are two ways of organizing difference. When differences are not too different, the system can do the work of integration without too much difficulty, and the system can change from simple to more complex without too many growing pains. When differences are too different, the system will either close its boundaries and keep the differences out or let the difference in, but keep it split off from the rest of the system so that it doesn't upset the system. Sometimes the system maintains the split, and whatever developmental potential would have developed from integrating the difference is lost permanently. Other times, as the system develops greater sophistication, the difference is then taken in and integrated.

Systems change and transform by integrating difference. The give and take of unfamiliar information between the system and its environment requires both the system and its environment to develop the ability to change. Differences make for bad relationships within the system and between the system and its environment in the short run, but in the long run, integrating differences are what contributes to system change and transformation

The process of transformation depends upon system recognition and integration of both similarities and differences – differences in the apparently similar and similarities in the apparently different. Organizing and integrating new information leads to transformations of living human systems from simpler to ever more complex in both structure and function.[5]

Definition of structure

The definition of structure is that every system is defined by its boundaries in space, time, reality and role. Boundaries in space and time are the structural elements common to all the systems in the hierarchy. The state of the group boundaries determine the energy that is contained within the group for the work the group needs to do to reach its goals.

Boundaries exist both in real time and space and in psychological time and space. Geographical space boundaries mark the threshold between the system inside and outside. Boundaries in clock time differentiate between the past, present and the future. Psychological space and time is like the time and space travel of the mind. In the imagination it is possible to travel from the present to the past or the future, from awareness of the here-and-now group, to imaginations about the here-and-now group.

Boundaries are permeable. Communications between one system and all other systems in the hierarchy have to cross the boundaries. This is the same as whether the hierarchy is within an individual system, or a group system, or between systems. The goldfish in the Introduction are a good analogy for this: the word goldfish can represent a single goldfish, a subgroup of goldfish or the shoal of goldfish, depending on the level of abstraction.[6]

What governs communication within, between and among systems is the permeability of boundaries and what influences the permeability of boundaries is noise in the communication. Systems close their boundaries to noisy communications and open them to clear communications. Shannon and Weaver (1964), in developing their information theory, had discovered that ambiguities, contradictions and redundancies in a message acted like noise in the communication channel and made it less likely that the information contained in the communication would get across.[7]

There appeared to be two kinds of problems in communication that had to be solved. First of all, the problem of *how* to communicate without introducing unnecessary noise into the system, and second, *what* to communicate that would solve the problems that the group had come to solve. Solving the problems of how to communicate was obviously a more fundamental problem, in that it would affect whether or not what was being communicated would be heard (Agazarian 1989b).

Confronted with the issue of boundary permeability, the issue was not only how to clear up the noise in the communication *after* it had entered the group but *before*: in other words, to influence the nature of the communication *at the boundary* (Agazarian 1992).

This was a challenging task. Another important building block in SAVI theory was Lewin's force field (Lewin 1951) of driving and restraining forces which I saw as synonymous with the approach and avoidance categories in the SAVI map. If I put the idea of Lewin's idea of driving and restraining forces together with Shannon and Weaver's (1964) definition of noise, it became a simple theoretical matter of weakening the ambiguities, redundancies and contradictions both at the boundaries of the system and also in the communication pattern within the system.

The method of boundarying

The method that I developed to reduce the restraining forces at the boundary was 'The Hierarchy of Defense Modification.' As I experimented with defense modification in the group I discovered that, just as there were specific communication patterns that typified the different phases of group development, so there were specific clusters of defenses that characterized each phase: thus the *hierarchy* of defense modification. As I continued to experiment with modifying the defenses that seemed generic to each phase and subphase, it also became clear that these very defenses were also the restraining forces to the development from one phase to another, and that by weakening the defensive restraining forces, the inherent drive was released, and the system moved towards the goals of survival, development and transformation from simpler to more complex, as defined in a theory of living human systems.

In other words, through the method of boundarying, the system was in a state to *function* in relation to its goals. I was already developing techniques for blocking the noise in communication at the boundary of the system (the distraction exercise); now the challenge was to address the noise inside the boundaries. Learning how to communicate is learning not only to reduce the noise by reducing the potential for noise before it starts, but also for reducing the noise that is inherent in the process of communication.

Anyone who has tried to explain theory, for example, knows that it takes many different attempts before the person you are communicating to starts to understand what you are saying. This is true, not only in trying to communicate something difficult, but in any communication. It takes processing before a message is received, heard and understood. It takes the ability to discriminate the differences in what was apparently similar to what one is already thinking as well as the similarities in what is apparently different. Once these differences are discriminated, they must be integrated if the communication is not going to slide away as if it never happened. Communication is the bridge between structure and function.[8]

Boundaries exist in time, space and role. In that a role is a system, it contains energy, and its structure and function is similar to all other system roles. Each role system exists as a subsystem in the context of a larger system (for example, the SCT role of member) and the system role energy can be directed towards or away from the goals of the system. As the context changes, so do the goals. Thus role functions change as the context changes.

Groups survive by maintaining a predictable set of role relationships, change by developing new potential relationships and transform by integrating the potential for change. Stereotype roles fixate a group and functional roles develop the group.

Every group is made up of a specific constellation of roles, and the constellation changes as the group moves through the phases and subphases of group development. The dynamics of the group in each phase stimulate different role responses in group members. For example, the flight phase elicits volunteers for the role of identified patient, the fight phase elicits volunteers for the role of scapegoat. However, although many members may volunteer for the role, few are chosen – it is the group dynamics that determine whether or not a member will repeat an old role in the group or whether he or she will have to develop a new set of role responses. This is the power of group therapy.

The same role can serve as a driving force in one developmental context and as a restraining force in another. For example, compliant roles in the flight phase are a driving force as it is easier to establish group norms in a compliant group. In the fight phase, however, where it is important for the group to challenge norms, the compliant role becomes a restraining force.

In SCT, there is a deliberate 'freezing and unfreezing' of role constellations. Crossing the boundary between one phase and another requires shifting roles from the constellation that stabilized the previous phase into the constellation that will stabilize the new phase. Roles contain the dynamics of the group. Acting out these dynamics is a restraining force to group development, exploring the impulses to act out the role dynamics are driving forces to the development of the member, the subgroups and the group-as-a-whole.

Theoretically, roles have all the characteristic of a living human system: they have clear boundaries (it is the predictable pattern of behavior that defines a role). For example, the boundaries of the identified patient role system are different from the boundaries of the scapegoat role system – each set are permeable to some communications from the group and impermeable to others. Role boundaries separate the role system from the group system. Thus the group boundaries are permeable to some role communications and impermeable to others. Roles have an identifiable function (there is a characteristic pattern to the kinds of information that is discriminated and integrated into a role system) and they fit into an implicit hierarchy (maladaptive roles into a network of one-up or one-down role relationships, adaptive roles into a shifting hierarchy based on resources which emerge and submerge again in relation to the requirements of the group work).

Before I developed a theory of living human systems, I used role as the bridge construct between the dynamics of groups and the dynamics of individuals (Agazarian and Peters 1981). Now, I conceptualize roles as interactive subsystems of a system that has a common goal. All role systems are therefore isomorphic (similar in structure and function) and the potential for role system development is different in different contexts (Agazarian 1989a and 1989b).

The definition of function

The definition of function is that systems survive, develop and transform from simple to complex through the process of discriminating and integrating differences: differences in the apparently similar and similarities in the apparently different (Agazarian 1996b).

The way each system functions is similar to every other system in the hierarchy in that each system survives, develops from simple to more complex by managing appropriate boundary permeability to communication transactions within, between and among systems in the hierarchy; opens to information that is similar enough to be integrated and closes to information that is too different; and transforms through the dynamic principle of discriminating and integrating differences.[9]

The system potential for relating to its primary and secondary goals[10] is dependent upon the system's ability to recognize and integrate *both* similarities and differences: differences in the apparently similar and similarities in the apparently different. Survival, development and transformation are the primary goals inherent in all living human systems. Living human systems maintain themselves in relationship to their primary goals of survival, development and transformation by containing, discriminating and integrating information within and across their boundaries. Environmental mastery is the secondary goal generic to all living human systems and can be congruent or incongruent with system primary goals.

Operationally, differences in an SCT group are managed by the method of functional subgrouping.

There was a major stumbling block in trying to put into practice the functional definition that systems survive, develop and transform through the discrimination and integration of differences. This was fine conceptually, but in the real world human beings hate differences.

In groups, much of group behavior seems to manage the hatred of differences.[11] The polite, social behavior glosses over them, the vague, ambiguous or redundant communications hide them in a smoke screen, and the 'Yes, but…' communications conceal a disagreement and import a contradiction. Dynamically, differences in groups are either institutionalized, as in the election of an identified patient, or scapegoated. All this I knew already from thinking about my work in groups. The major challenge was how to influence the way groups function so that they could integrate differences rather than scapegoat them.

The answer came from one of the implications in the definition of hierarchy. The definition reads: 'Every system exists in the environment of the system above it and is the environment of the system below it.' As I have already mentioned, having defined the hierarchy as the member, subgroup and group-as-a-whole it was axiomatic that the subgroup existed in the environment of the group and was the environment for its members. This had revolutionized my understanding of group. It had not only added the dimension of the subgroup as a significant dynamic process to those already defined for the group and individual members, but it had also manifested as a fulcrum system whose boundaries it shared with both members and the group-as-a-whole. The implication was that probably the most effective point of application for influencing change was the subgroup, not the individual member or the group-as-a-whole itself.

The method of functional subgrouping

Functional subgrouping is a method for discriminating and integrating differences instead of stereotyping or scapegoating them. Functional subgroups come together around similarities instead of separating around difference. By exploring the differences in the apparently similar within each subgroup and the similarities in the apparently different between each subgroup, differences are contained and integrated in the system of the group-as-a-whole.

Functional subgrouping puts into practice the dynamic that SCT uses to explain the survival, development and transformation of living human systems: the ability to discriminate and integrate differences instead of stereotyping or scapegoating them. In subgrouping, rather than stereotyping, rejecting and scapegoating differences in self or other, conflicts around difference are taken out of the person and contained in the group. Within each subgroup, as the similarities among members are explored, so differences become apparent and accepted. As each subgroup in the group-as-a-whole recognizes differences in what is apparently similar within their subgroups, so they start to recognize similarities in what was apparently different between the subgroups, and so there is an integration in the group-as-a-whole.

It is clear that subgrouping exists all the time in a group and serves an important function in keeping the group stable – both implicit stereotype subgrouping, and also implicit functional subgrouping (when members spontaneously join around themes that are important to the dynamics or the task of the group) (Agazarian 1987, 1989a). The method of functional subgrouping explicitly and deliberately encourages subgrouping so that conflicts are contained in the group-as-a-whole in different subgroups, rather than acted out as conflicts between members or contained in stereotype subgroups. Thus, in an SCT group, functional subgrouping competes with the predictable impulse to establish a stabilizing group hierarchy based on stereotype (Agazarian 1997).

In stereotype subgrouping members come together around obvious similarities like race, religion and gender, thus establishing a group hierarchy based on one-up/one-down status rather than on resources. This leads easily into converting or scapegoating any member who does not conform. A status hierarchy is reinforced by stereotype communications at all system levels: in the member; between the members; in the subgroup; between the subgroups; and in the group-as-a-whole. (This is discussed at greater length in the Introduction). The major implication of the contrast between stereotype and functional subgrouping is that stereotype subgrouping is one of the restraining forces that systems-centered methods expect to modify, and functional subgrouping one of the driving forces that systems-centered methods expect to promote.

Definition of energy

Living human systems are energy organizing: system energy is organized and directed towards the goals of survival, development and environmental mastery by reducing the noise in the communications within, between and among all the different living human systems in the hierarchy of systems.

Theoretically, energy is assumed to be the 'force' that discriminates between living and non-living systems. It is assumed that living human systems survive, develop and transform by organizing and re-organizing energy.

Energy exists as actual or potential, organized or disorganized. Miller (1978) states that system drive energy can be equated with information: the potential and actual organization of energy or information in relationship to the goal. Thus, energy and information are synonymous – it is the discrimination and integration of information (energy) that enables the system to move towards its goals of survival, development and transformation. In SCT the force field (adapted from Lewin 1951) is used to picture how energy or information is organized in a system and how much energy is available for goal-oriented work.

Living human systems are energy organizing, self-correcting and goal-directed. They maintain communications between their internal organization of information and their external environment so that they can organize their energy and orient themselves towards the explicit and so implicit goals can be corrected. There are always problems to be solved along the path to goal, and systems are split between approaching them or avoiding them. This inherent approach/avoidance conflict is conceptualized in terms of a force field of driving and restraining forces. When the restraining forces are weakened the inherent drive towards the goal is released. Living human systems can acquire the ability to weaken their own restraining forces, and thus re-orient in the goal direction.

The force field is a model of the driving and restraining forces that maintain the equilibrium of a system between the drive to maintain stability and the drive to change. Lewin (1951) introduced the model of the force field to diagnose the relationship between the system and a defined goal, and demonstrated that it was more efficient and effective to weaken the restraining forces on the path to the goal than it was to increase the driving forces. Building on his work, I redefined the forces in his force field (Agazarian 1988) as vectors, and thus both the driving and restraining forces were related to a goal. This enabled me to define the restraining forces as defenses and the driving forces as the inherent drive towards the goals of survival, development and transformation.

The method of vectoring

A vector is like an arrow which has velocity, a direction and a target. This definition (borrowed from physics) is an excellent descriptor for the driving and restraining forces of a force field.

Vectoring is the method which directs the energy in the hierarchy of systems, and connects the system roles to the system goals. Vectoring is the word to describe the process that enables members deliberately to choose to direct their energy towards the aspects of themselves that they want to learn more about, and deliberately to direct their energy away from the defenses and symptoms that interfere with their curiosity. Learning how to vector their energy also increases members' ability to direct their energy away from the fantasies and fears about the past, present and future into the reality of the here-and-now. Vectoring also makes it possible for members to focus their energy outside themselves so that they can join a subgroup. Both in subgrouping and boundarying, people learn that if they don't give energy to their defenses, symptoms, distractions, negative predictions and mind-readings, they not only have plenty of energy available to direct towards testing their reality, but they also do not generate the defenses and symptoms that exhaust their energy.

Vectoring interventions make working goals explicit so that the energy of the group-as-a-whole, the subgroups and the members can be redirected towards the work of the group.

In SCT, avoiding weakening defensive restraining forces before the system is ready to make the change required to function without them is managed by following the hierarchy of defense modification which requires weakening only those restraining forces appropriate to the context of the phase of group development. Thus the inherent driving forces towards survival, development and transformation are released, which are synonymous with the goals of therapy.

Summary

In systems-centered therapy, communications, within, between and among living human systems at all system levels, in the hierarchy of member, subgroup and the group-as-a-whole, are influenced through the methods of contextualizing and vectoring, boundarying and functional subgrouping. Boundarying makes the boundaries permeable to information through the techniques of the hierarchy of defense modification. Functional subgrouping manages the process of discrimination and integration by bypassing the conflict in the individual members and containing it in the group-as-a-whole, while the different sides of the conflict are discriminated and integrated, first within subgroups and then between subgroups. Vectoring connects the group energy to the goals of survival, development and transformation. Contextualizing brings about the systems-centered group by developing the consciousness of the member, subgroup and group-as-a-whole. This in turn develops the capacity of the members to experience themselves as self-centered systems in a systems-centered context.

It is one of my goals for SCT that, when systems-centered therapists make interventions in a systems-centered therapy, each intervention tests a hypothesis developed from constructs of a theory of living human systems. Then, if the intervention influences the system's movement towards the goals of therapy in the predicted direction, the theory has been supported. If it doesn't, then the research question becomes what made the difference this time, in this context. A good example of how this is made operational is in the research question at the end of the boundarying 'distraction exercise.' The distraction exercise is designed to bring the person's energy across the boundary from the environment into the here-and-now of the group. This is tested each time by the research question that ends it: 'Are you more here, less here or the same?'

And this is a good question with which to end this book.

Notes

1   The concept of Lewin's (1951) life space is a good transition into what I mean. Lewin thought about people's perception of their environment in terms of a map which he called a life space. He assumed that if one could read a person's map, one could predict how he would behave. 'Perception now,' he wrote, 'is behavior next.'

2   Discriminating between thinking and emotion is the first step in developing three subgroups to explore in the self (and with others) – the thinking or comprehensive subsystem, the emotional or apprehensive subsystem, and the observing subsystem that discriminates and integrates the two kinds of information into two different kinds of knowledge – comprehension and apprehension.

3   Similarities and differences in the hierarchy of living systems are communicated across system boundaries. Systems exist in a hierarchy of similarities and differences. System boundaries are open to similarities but often closed to difference. Similarities are already familiar to the system's internal organization, and do not introduce the system to much that is new. Systems let in the familiar with little difficulty. Integrating similarities does not require the system to change.

Systems survive by developing internal organizing principles to manage the information in communications within, between and among the system hierarchy.

Systems stay stable and survive by integrating similarities. Give and take of familiar information between the system and its environment maintain the system in a good relationship with its inner and outer world, keep the system stable and increase the probability that it will survive in the short run. Too much similarity and not enough difference, however, introduces redundancy and rigidity, which in the long run will threaten the system survival.

4   It was a great challenge when I reached this stage in developing the theory. If I could define structure and function clearly enough I could develop methods and techniques that would also work for the member, a subgroup or the group-as-a-whole.

5   Dynamically, system transformation is a function of the process of discriminating and integrating the information contained in the communication transactions that cross the boundaries between, within and among systems in the hierarchy. System transformation is determined by its ability to remain in equilibrium during the process (containing the chaos of unintegrated information – often called the unconscious).

6   I had used Shannon and Weaver's information theory (1964) as an important building block when I developed SAVI (system for analyzing verbal interaction) with my friend Anita Simon (Simon and Agazarian 1967). SAVI has been invaluable in being able to

draw a map of the communication pattern of the group, or the individual, collecting the data in a three by three grid, the rows of which identified the approach or avoidance character of the communication and the rows identifying whether the communication was predominantly personal, factual, or orienting. What the communications approached or avoided was the problems that inevitably lie on the path to a goal. (This building block came from Howard and Scott's theory of stress (1965).)

Applying SAVI to group communication, I had learned a lot about the kinds of communication patterns that typify the phases of group development. I used Bennis and Shepard's (1957) model of group development, and developed a communication pattern for subphases, like flight and fight, that they define. This then enabled me to intervene within a clear frame, attempting to reduce the avoidance behaviors and increase the approach behaviors *once the communication was set.*

7   Shannon and Weaver (1964) also discover that the formula that they developed for reducing 'noise' in a communication channel was the reciprocal of the entropy formula in the second law of thermodynamics. Thus, information exists on a continuum of organization from too organized (redundant or rigid) to too disorganized (ambiguous).

8   Boundarying increases the appropriate permeability of boundaries so that system energy (information) – by systematically and sequentially reducing defenses and symptoms – increases the permeability of the boundaries to communications which contain the energy that relates to the goals. Boundarying enables members to focus their attention away from their past into the here-and-now and deal with the defenses that prevent them from being who they want to be, and saying what they want to say, in the group. By boundarying, people learn to recognize how they leave their here-and-now reality and emigrate across the boundaries of space and time. People leave in two ways: in reality by changing locations or by ignoring clock time; in psychological reality by turning their thoughts and emotions towards the past or the future, or by leaving the here-and-now experience and living in the reality created by their thoughts.

9   Integration and survival, development and transformation are the primary goals of living systems to which the change energy is directed. Changes occur within, between and among all systems and subsystems in the hierarchy through communication exchanges across the boundaries. Communication transactions require the system to discriminate and integrate information, both information that requires discriminations of difference in the apparently similar, and of similarities in the apparently different. Integration of this information requires the system to de-stabilize and re-stabilize in an ongoing, self-correcting process that transforms the system on the one hand, and on the other relates the system to its primary goals of survival, development and transformation.

10   How the system functions in relationship to these goals will, however, be different in different contexts.

11   Pat de Maré (1991) says that it is through the metabolization of hatred that creativity in a group arises.

References

Agazarian, Y.M. (1969) 'A Theory of Verbal Behavior and Information Transfer.' *Classroom Interaction Newsletter 4*, 2, 22–33

Agazarian, Y.M. (1982) 'Role as a Bridge Construct in Understanding the Relationship Between the Individual and the Group.' In M. Pines and L. Rafaelson (eds) *The Individual and the Group, Boundaries and Interrelations. Volume I: Theory.* New York: Plenum Press.

Agazarian, Y.M. (1986) 'Application of Lewin's Life Space Concept to the Individual and Group-as-a-Whole Systems in Psychotherapy.' In E. Stivers and S. Wheelan (eds) *The Lewin Legacy: Field Theory in Current Practice.* New York: Springer-Verlag.

Agazarian, Y.M. (1988) 'Application of a Modified Force Field Analysis to the Diagnosis of Implicit Group Goals.' Unpublished paper delivered at the Third International Kurt Lewin Conference, sponsored by the Society for the Advancement of Field Theory, September 1988.

Agazarian, Y.M. (1989a) 'The Invisible Group: An Integrational Theory of Group-as-a-Whole', the 12th Annual Foulkes Memorial Lecture. In *Group Analysis: The Journal of the Group Analytic Psychotherapy 22*, 4.

Agazarian, Y.M. (1989b) 'Group-as-a-Whole Systems Theory and Practice.' *Group: Special Issue on the Group-as-a-whole. Group: The Journal of the Eastern Group Psychotherapy Society 13*, 3, 4, 131–155.

Agazarian, Y.M. (1992) 'A Systems Approach to the Group-as-a-Whole.' *International Journal of Group Psychotherapy 42*, 3.

Agazarian, Y.M. (1993) 'Reframing the Group-as-a-Whole.' In T. Hugg, N. Carson, and T. Lipgar (eds) *Changing Group Relations: The Next Twenty-Five Years in America. Proceedings of the Ninth Scientific Meeting of the A.K. Rice Institute.* Jupiter, FL: AKRI Institute.

Agazarian, Y. (1994) 'The Phases of Development and the Systems-Centered Group.' In M. Pines and V. Schermer *Ring of Fire: Primitive Object Relations and Affect in Group Psychotherapy.* London: Routledge, Chapman and Hall.

Agazarian, Y.M. (1996) 'An Up-to-Date Guide to the Theory, Constructs and Hypotheses of a Theory of Living Human Systems and its Systems-Centered Practice.' In *The SCT Journal.* Philadelphia: Systems-Centered Press.

Agazarian, Y.M. (1997) *Systems-Centered Therapy for Groups.* New York: Guilford.

Agazarian, Y.M. (1999) 'Phases of Development in the Systems-Centered Group.' *Small Group Research 30*, 1, 82–107.

Agazarian, Y.M. and Janoff, S. (1993) 'Systems Theory and Small Groups.' In I. Kapplan and B. Sadock (eds) *Comprehensive Textbook of Group Psychotherapy* (3rd edition). Baltimore, MD: Williams and Wilkins.

Agazarian, Y.M. and Peters, R. (1981) *The Visible and Invisible Group: Two Perspectives on Group Psychotherapy and Group Process.* London: Routledge and Kegan Paul. (Reprinted in paperback 1987.)

Bennis, W.G. and Shepard, H. A. (1957). 'A Theory of Group Development.' *Human Relations 9*, 4, 415–437.

Bertalanffy, L. von (1969) *General Systems*. Revised edition. New York: George Braziller.

Bion, W.R. (1959) *Experiences in Groups*. London: Tavistock.

Davanloo, H. (1987) 'Clinical Manifestations of Superego Pathology.' *International Journal of Short-Term Psychotherapy 2*, 225–254.

de Maré, P., Piper R., and Thompson, S. (1991) *Koinonia: From Hate, through Dialogue, to Culture in the Large Group*. London: Karnac Books.

Durkin, H.E. (1964) *The Group in Depth*. New York: International Universities Press, Inc.

Goleman, D. (1995) *Emotional Intelligence*. New York: Bantam Books.

Howard, A. and Scott, R. A. (1965) 'A Proposed Framework for the Analysis of Stress in the Human Organism.' *Journal of Applied Behavioral Science 10*, 141–160.

Korzybski, A. (1948) *Science and Sanity: An Introduction to Non-Aristotelian Systems and General Semantics* (3rd edition). Lakeville, Conn: International Non-Aristotelian Library, Institute of General Semantics.

Lewin, K. (1951) *Field Theory in Social Science*. New York: Harper and Row.

Miller, J.G. (1978) *Living Systems*. New York: McGraw Hill.

Shannon, C.E. and Weaver, W. (1964) *The Mathematical Theory of Communication*. Urbana, IL: University of Illinois Press.

Simon, A. and Agazarian, Y.M. (1967) *SAVI: Sequential Analysis of Verbal Interaction*. Research for Better Schools, Philadelphia.

Simon, A. and Agazarian, Y.M. (2000) 'The System for Analyzing Verbal Interaction.' In *The Process of Group Psychotherapy: Systems for Analyzing Change*. Washington, DC: American Psychological Association.

Yalom, I., Liebermann, M., and Miles, M., (1973) *Encounter Groups: First Facts*. New York: Basic Books.

Subject Index

Name Index